BLADDER BIOPSY INTERPRETATION

Biopsy Interpretation Series

BIOPSY INTERPRETATION SERIES

Series Editor: Jonathan I. Epstein, M.D.

Prostate Biopsy Interpretation, Third Edition
Jonathan I. Epstein and Ximing J. Yang, 2002

Interpretation of Breast Biopsies, Fourth Edition
Darryl Carter, 2002

Biopsy Interpretation of the Liver
Stephen A. Geller and Lydia M. Petrovic, 2004

Bladder Biopsy Interpretation
Jonathan I. Epstein, Mahul B. Amin, and Victor E. Reuter, 2004

BLADDER BIOPSY INTERPRETATION

Biopsy Interpretation Series

Jonathan I. Epstein, M.D.

Director of Surgical Pathology
Professor, Departments of Pathology, Urology, and Oncology
The Reinhard Professor of Urological Pathology
The Johns Hopkins School of Medicine
Baltimore, Maryland

Mahul B. Amin, M.D.

Director of Surgical Pathology
Professor, Departments of Pathology, Urology, Hematology, and Oncology
Associate Director, Cancer Pathogenomics
Winship Cancer Institute
Emory University School of Medicine
Atlanta, Georgia

Victor E. Reuter, M.D.

Attending Pathologist
Memorial Hospital Member, Memorial Hospital
Memorial Sloan–Kettering Cancer Center
Professor of Pathology
Weill Medical College of Cornell University
New York, New York

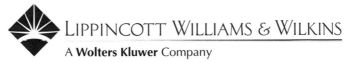

LIPPINCOTT WILLIAMS & WILKINS
A **Wolters Kluwer** Company
Philadelphia · Baltimore · New York · London
Buenos Aires · Hong Kong · Sydney · Tokyo

Acquisitions Editor: Ruth W. Weinberg
Developmental Editor: Lisa Consoli
Production Editor: Jonathan Geffner
Manufacturing Manager: Colin Warnock
Cover Designer: Karen Quigley
Compositor: Lippincott Williams & Wilkins Desktop Division
Printer: Maple Press

© 2004 by LIPPINCOTT WILLIAMS & WILKINS
530 Walnut Street
Philadelphia, PA 19106 USA
LWW.com

Library of Congress Cataloging-in-Publication Data

Epstein, Jonathan I.
    Bladder biopsy interpretation / Jonathan I. Epstein, Mahul B. Amin, Victor E. Reuter.
        p. ; cm.—(Biopsy interpretation series)
    Includes bibliographical references and index.
    ISBN 0-7817-4276-5
        1. Bladder—Tumors—Cytodiagnosis. 2. Bladder—Needle biopsy. 3. Bladder—Diseases—Cytodiagnosis. I. Amin, Mahul B. II. Reuter, Victor E. III. Title. IV. Series.
    [DNLM: 1. Bladder Neoplasms—pathology. WJ 504 E64b 2004]
    RC280.B5E67 2004
    616.6'20758—dc22
                                                                        2003058869

Care has been taken to confirm the accuracy of the information presented and to describe generally accepted practices. However, the authors and publisher are not responsible for errors or omissions or for any consequences from application of the information in this book and make no warranty, expressed or implied, with respect to the currency, completeness, or accuracy of the contents of the publication. Application of this information in a particular situation remains the professional responsibility of the practitioner.

The authors and publisher have exerted every effort to ensure that drug selection and dosage set forth in this text are in accordance with current recommendations and practice at the time of publication. However, in view of ongoing research, changes in government regulations, and the constant flow of information relating to drug therapy and drug reactions, the reader is urged to check the package insert for each drug for any change in indications and dosage and for added warnings and precautions. This is particularly important when the recommended agent is a new or infrequently employed drug.

Some drugs and medical devices presented in this publication have Food and Drug Administration (FDA) clearance for limited use in restricted research settings. It is the responsibility of the health care provider to ascertain the FDA status of each drug or device planned for use in their clinical practice.

10 9 8 7 6 5 4 3 2

Contents

Preface

Bladder Biopsy Interpretation includes, among many other advances, the modern principles of classification put forth in the 2003 World Health Organization "Blue Book." Our understanding of urologic pathology has undergone many changes during the last decade; and nowhere is this statement more valid than in urothelial diseases, particularly neoplasia. For example, a new grading classification has been adopted and its morphologic and cytologic criteria better defined. Variants of urothelial carcinoma have been defined, some with distinct clinical characteristics. The microanatomy of the urothelium and bladder wall has been expanded and criteria for establishing the presence and depth of invasion further refined, leading to improved correlation between stage and clinical outcome. In addition, we now have markers that help establish the diagnosis of urothelial cancer and may help us predict outcome, together with morphology. Nonneoplastic conditions are discussed with equal detail.

A major feature of this book is the accompanying CD-ROM, which contains over 1,200 color images. In the book, we are unable to illustrate the full spectrum of morphologic features of any given entity. The CD-ROM allows us to illustrate multiple color images of each entity at different magnifications. Together with the text, these illustrations will enhance the educational experience leading to a greater level of diagnostic confidence.

Bladder Biopsy Interpretation and the accompanying CD-ROM focus on state-of-the-art, practical information that is required to properly evaluate biopsies of the urothelial tract. Much has been learned about the molecular events associated with the development and progression of urothelial carcinoma; however, at this time, this information has proven of marginal utility in clinical practice. Consequently, the molecular aspects of this disease are not covered in any detail. This situation is certain to change in the future, and this fact will be reflected in future editions.

Jonathan I. Epstein, M.D.
Mahul B. Amin, M.D.
Victor E. Reuter, M.D.

Acknowledgments

Dr. Amin acknowledges the secretarial assistance of his administrative assistant Suzzane Briceno (for manuscript typing and preparation).

Dr. Epstein acknowledges Dr. Rolondo Milord, who took excellent photographs of many of the color images within the CD-ROM while he was a fellow in urological pathology at The Johns Hopkins Hospital; and his Administrative Assistant, Janet Muller, for her help in preparing the manuscript.

Dr. Reuter acknowledges the assistance of his Administrative Assistant, Maureen Flaherty, in the preparation and editing of this manuscript.

1

Normal Bladder Anatomy and Variants of Normal Histology

The epithelium of the urinary bladder and urethra is entirely derived from endoderm of the urogenital sinus, whereas the lamina propria, muscularis propria, and adventitia develop from the surrounding splanchnic mesenchyme. Despite their different histogenesis, all of the urinary excretory passages are lined by so-called transitional epithelium, which is better referred to as *urothelium*, a term that is used throughout this text. During early embryologic development, the caudal portions of the mesonephric ducts contribute to the formation of the mucosa of the bladder trigone but are eventually replaced by endoderm (1).

The wall of the urinary bladder is formed of four layers: (a) urothelium, (b) lamina propria, (c) muscularis propria, and (d) adventitia or serosa (Fig. 1.1) (efigs 1–5). Depending on the location, these layers may be surrounded by perivesical fat (2,3). The thickness of the urothelium varies, as does the shape of the epithelial cells, depending on the degree to which the bladder is distended. In the empty bladder, the epithelium can be up to seven cells thick. The deepest (basal) cells have a cuboidal or columnar shape, above which are several layers of irregularly polyhedral cells. The most superficial or luminal layer consists of large, sometimes binucleated cells with abundant eosinophilic cytoplasm and a rounded free surface. They are descriptively called *umbrella* or *superficial cells* (2). In the distended bladder, the epithelial lining can be as few as two cells thick, with a basal layer of cuboidal cells and a superficial layer of elongated and flattened umbrella cells (see Chapter 2 for histology of normal urothelium).

A thin basement membrane separates the urothelium from the underlying lamina propria. The latter is formed of abundant connective tissue containing a rich vascular network, lymphatic channels, sensory nerve endings, and a few elastic fibers. The lamina propria varies in thickness in the empty versus the distended bladder, but is generally thinner in the areas of the trigone and bladder neck. Wisps or small fascicles of smooth muscle may be found within the superficial lamina propria, either isolated or forming a complete or incomplete muscularis mucosae (3,4) (Fig. 1.2) (efigs 5–9). This muscularis mucosae, if present, is fre-

1

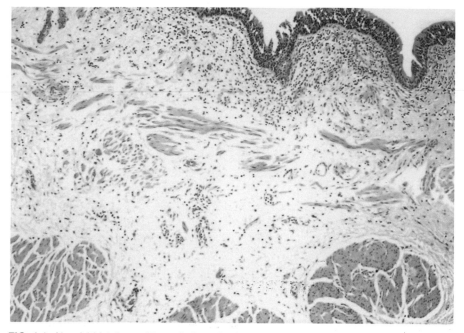

FIG. 1.1. Normal histology with urothelium, lamina propria, muscularis mucosae, submucosa, and muscularis propria.

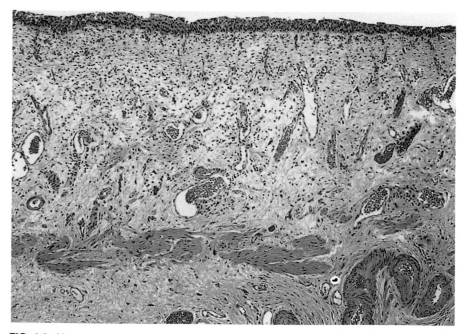

FIG. 1.2. Normal histology with urothelium, lamina propria, muscularis mucosae, submucosa, and muscularis propria.

quently seen in association with medium-sized vessels, which are also prominently seen within the lamina propria (Fig. 1.3). It must not be confused with the smooth muscle bundles of the muscularis propria because this might result in errors of tumor staging and treatment. There may be fat within the lamina propria as well as in the muscularis propria (5) (Fig. 1.4) (efigs 10–12). Fat may be found in bladders that have never been instrumented or in areas of prior transurethral resection. Whether the presence of fat is due to a normal anatomic variant, a function of the patient's body habitus, or a metaplastic phenomenon is not known. What is important is that the presence of invasive tumor at the level of smooth muscle or fat in a transurethral resection specimen does not necessarily warrant a diagnosis of muscularis propria invasion or extravesical extension.

The muscularis propria, also known as detrusor muscle, has loosely anastomosing, ill-defined internal and external longitudinal layers and a more prominent middle circular layer of muscle (efigs 13–18). The bundles of muscle seen at this site are generally much larger than those present in the lamina propria, a feature that is useful as an anatomic landmark (Fig. 1.5). In the bladder neck of the male, the fascicles of the muscularis propria are continuous with the fibromuscular tissue of the prostate (2). As previously mentioned, fat may be present between the muscle bundles of the muscularis propria. The outermost layer of the viscus is an adventitia of connective tissue; only the superior surface is covered by serosa of the pelvic peritoneum.

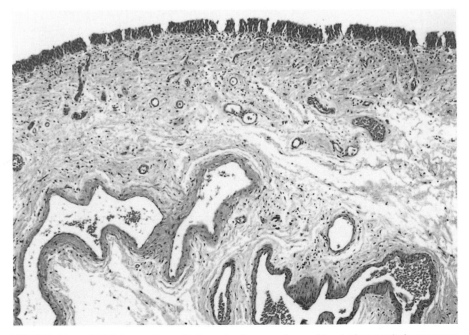

FIG. 1.3. Normal histology with urothelium, lamina propria, and level of muscularis mucosae associated with numerous prominent blood vessels.

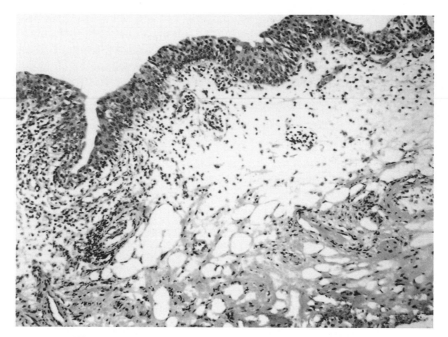

FIG. 1.4. Normal histology with adipose tissue in lamina propria.

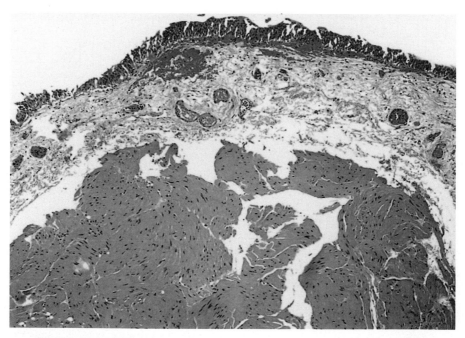

FIG. 1.5. Muscularis propria (detrusor muscle) extending close to mucosal surface.

The adult empty bladder has the shape of a four-sided inverted pyramid and is enveloped by the vesical fascia (6). The superior surface faces superiorly and is covered by the pelvic parietal peritoneum. The posterior surface, also known as the base of the bladder, faces posteriorly and inferiorly. It is separated from the rectum by the uterine cervix and the proximal portions of the vagina in females and by the seminal vesicles and the ampulla of the vasa deferentia in males. These posterior anatomic relationships are clinically important. Because most bladder neoplasms arise in the posterior wall adjacent to the ureteral orifices, invasive tumor may extend into adjacent soft tissue and organs. The intimate relationships to the previously mentioned organs account for why hysterectomy and partial vaginectomy are indicated at the time of radial cystectomy in women. Conversely, seminal vesicle involvement is a bad prognostic sign in bladder carcinoma in males, a reflection of high pathologic stage.

The bladder bed (structures on which the bladder neck rests) is formed posteriorly by the rectum in males and vagina in females. Anteriorly and laterally it is formed by the internal obturator and levator ani muscles as well as the pubic bones. These structures may be involved in advanced tumors occupying the anterior, lateral, or bladder neck regions and render the patient inoperable.

The most anterosuperior point of the bladder is called the *apex* or *dome* and is located at the point of contact of the superior surfaces and the two inferolateral surfaces. The apex marks the point of insertion of the median umbilical ligament and consequently is the area where urachal carcinomas occur.

VARIANTS OF NORMAL HISTOLOGY

One important feature of urothelium is its ability to transform its morphologic appearance, most likely as a reaction to a local stimulus (usually some sort of injury). The end result is that urothelium may take on a host of benign morphologic features that are so common that they are considered variants of normal histology.

Von Brunn Nests

The most common reactive proliferative change within the urothelium is the formation of von Brunn nests, which represent invaginations of the surface urothelium into the underlying lamina propria (7–10) (Fig. 1.6) (efigs 19, 20). Basal and intermediate cells are readily identifiable. In some cases, these solid nests of benign-appearing urothelium may lose continuity with the surface, becoming isolated within the superficial lamina propria. Such proliferations may mimic the nested variant of urothelial carcinoma, particularly if the nests lie relatively deep in the lamina propria. In contrast to nested variant of urothelial carcinoma, examples of florid von Brunn nests in the bladder generally show larger nests with more regular shapes and regular spacing (11) (Figs. 1.7, 1.8). In florid von Brunn nests, cyst formation is more pronounced and involves a higher pro-

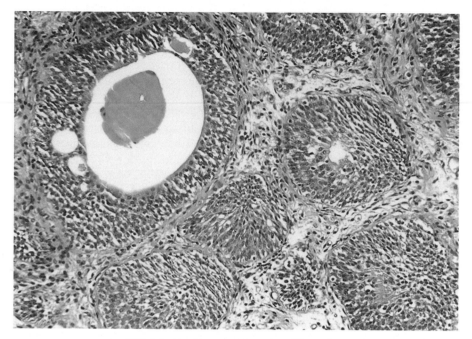

FIG. 1.6. Von Brunn nests and cystitis cystica.

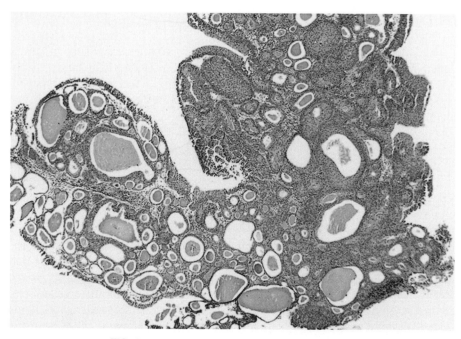

FIG. 1.7. Florid cystitis cystica with cystic dilatation.

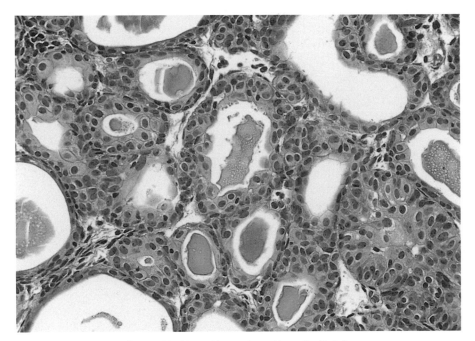

FIG. 1.8. Florid cystitis cystica with cystic dilatation.

portion of nest structures; apical glandular differentiation and eosinophilic secretions are also more common, acquiring features of cystitis cystica and cystitis glandularis (see later discussion). Atypia is absent, and the lesions have a flat noninfiltrative base. Cases of florid von Brunn nests in the ureter may show small nests similar to nested variant of urothelial carcinoma (Figs. 1.9, 1.10). Distinguishing features in florid von Brunn nests include a flat noninfiltrative base, a lobular or linear array of the nests, and a lack of cytologic atypia. Wide variation in staining for MIB-1, p53, p27, and cytokeratin 20 is seen in both florid von Brunn nests and nested variant of urothelial carcinoma, such that, except in a few cases, a specific cutoff value cannot be determined for diagnostic purposes (11).

Cystitis Cystica and Cystitis Glandularis

The term *cystitis cystica* has been coined to describe when the nests become cystically dilated, acquiring a luminal space (Figs. 1.11, 1.12) (efigs 21–27). Some cases of von Brunn nests, cystitis cystica, or cystitis glandularis may mimic invasive urothelial carcinoma (efigs 28–54). In this setting, the umbrella cell layer may take on a cuboidal or columnar appearance. In some cases, the epithelial lining undergoes glandular metaplasia, giving rise to what is called cystitis glandularis (Fig. 1.11) (12). The cells become cuboidal or columnar and

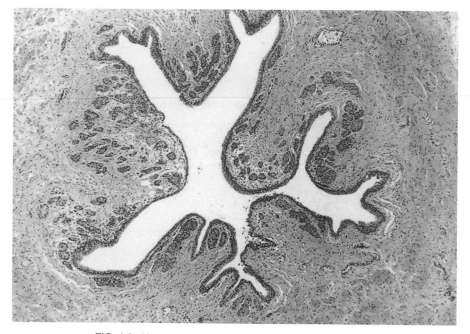

FIG. 1.9. Ureter with florid proliferation of von Brunn nests.

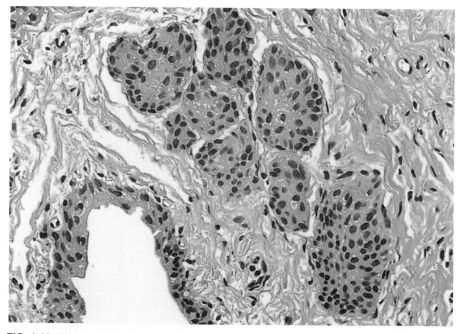

FIG. 1.10. Ureter with florid proliferation of von Brunn nests (high magnification of Figure 1.9).

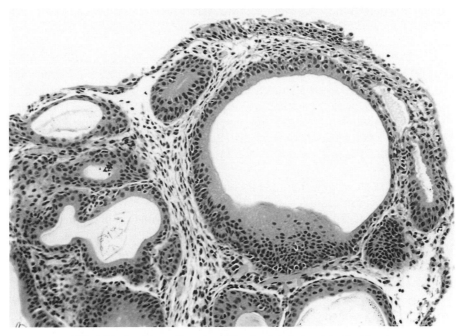

FIG. 1.11. Cystitis cystica et cystitis glandularis (nonintestinal type).

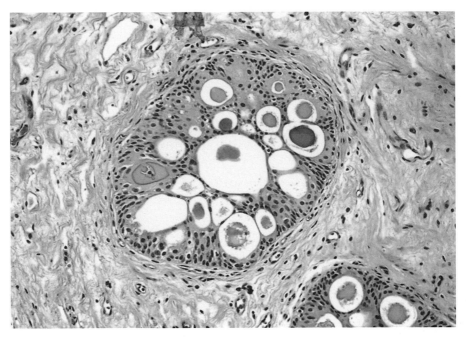

FIG. 1.12. Cystitis cystica.

mucin secreting. If the epithelium acquires intestinal-type goblet cells, this variant is called *cystitis glandularis with intestinal metaplasia* (colonic metaplasia) (see Chapter 8).

von Brunn nests, cystitis cystica, and cystitis glandularis represent a continuum of proliferative or reactive changes seen along the entire urothelial tract, and it is common to see all three in the same specimen. Most investigators believe that they occur as a result of local inflammatory insult (7,8). Nevertheless, these proliferative changes are seen in the urothelium of patients with no evidence of local inflammation so that it is possible that they also represent either normal histologic variants or the residual effects of an old inflammatory process (9,10).

Much has been written about the association of von Brunn nests, cystitis cystica, and especially cystitis glandularis and urothelial carcinoma (7–14). The high incidence of these proliferative changes in normal bladder suggests that they are not likely premalignant changes and that there is no cause-effect relationship between their presence and the appearance of bladder cancer. It is true that one or all of these changes are commonly present in biopsy specimens containing bladder cancer, but the coexistence may be coincidental or the cancer itself may be producing the local inflammatory insult that causes them and not vice versa. The fact that exceptional cases may occur in which carcinoma clearly arises within the epithelium of these reactive lesions does not alter this argument (13,14).

REFERENCES

1. Moore KL. *The developing human*, 3rd ed. Philadelphia: WB Saunders, 1982:267.
2. Fawcett DW. *Bloom and Fawcett: a textbook of histology*, 11th ed. Philadelphia: WB Saunders 1986:787–790.
3. Reuter VE. Urinary bladder and ureter. In: Sternberg SS, ed. *Histology for pathologists*, 2nd ed. New York: Raven Press, 1997:835–847.
4. Ro JY, Ayala AG, El-Naggar A. Muscularis mucosa of urinary bladder: importance for staging and treatment. *Am J Surg Pathol* 1987;11:668–673.
5. Philip AT, Amin MB, Tamboli P, et al. Intravesical adipose tissue. Quantitative study of its presence and location with implications for therapy and prognosis. *Am J Surg Pathol* 2000;24:1286–1290.
6. Moore KL. *Clinically oriented anatomy*, 2nd ed. Baltimore: Williams & Wilkins, 1985:265.
7. Morse HD. The etiology and pathology of pyelitis cystica, ureteritis cystica and cystitis cystica. *Am J Pathol* 1928;4:33–50.
8. Mostofi FK. Potentialities of bladder epithelium. *J Urol* 1954;71:705–714.
9. Goldstein AMB, Fauer RB, Chinn M, et al. New concepts on formation of Brunn's nests and cysts in the urinary tract mucosa. *Urology* 1978;11:513–517.
10. Wiener DP, Koss LG, Sablay B, et al. The prevalence and significance of Brunn's nests, cystitis cystica and squamous metaplasia in normal bladders. *J Urol* 1979;122:317–321.
11. Volmar KE, Chan TY, De Marzo AM, et al. Florid von Brunn nests mimicking urothelial carcinoma: a morphologic and immunohistochemical comparison to the nested variant of urothelial carcinoma. *Am J Surg Pathol* 2003;27:1243–1252.
12. Davies G, Castro JE. Cystitis glandularis. *Urology* 1977;10:128–129.
13. Edwards PD, Hurm RA, Jaeschke WH. Conversion of cystitis glandularis to adenocarcinoma. *J Urol* 1972;108:568–580.
14. Lin JI, Tseng CH, Choy C, et al. Diffuse cystitis glandularis associated with adenocarcinomatous change. *Urology* 1980;15:411–415.

2

Flat Urothelial Lesions

There are four main reasons a surgical pathologist is asked to evaluate flat (cystoscopically apparent or unapparent) lesions. The first two indications involve multiple random biopsies by cold cup biopsy technique (a) in patients previously diagnosed with noninvasive or lamina propria–invasive papillary tumors who are on surveillance for bladder cancer and (b) in patients given the diagnosis of papillary bladder cancer for the first time. The aim of the biopsies is to detect flat intraurothelial disease, which suggests urothelial instability, multifocality, and proclivity for disease progression. The third indication is in patients with hematuria, dysuria, and increased frequency of micturition, who either have positive urine cytology or are at high risk of development of bladder cancer. The aim is to detect urothelial carcinoma in situ (CIS), which may or may not be cystoscopically apparent. The fourth indication is in patients without a high risk of bladder cancer but who present with urinary symptoms similar to those listed but who do not respond to routine medical treatments. In this setting, biopsies are performed to evaluate other causes for the symptoms.

APPROACH TO THE DIAGNOSIS OF FLAT LESIONS

The World Health Organization (WHO)/International Society of Urological Pathology (ISUP) classification of flat intraurothelial lesions is outlined in Table 2.1 (1). Because WHO has accepted the nomenclature used for flat lesions used in WHO/ISUP (1998) in its entirety, the system is currently referred to as WHO(2003)/ISUP. The approach to the diagnosis of lesions within this classification requires attention to several organizational and cytologic features within the urothelium, the constellation of the presence or absence of which helps make the correct diagnosis (2) (Table 2.2).

Attention to the thickness of the urothelium may provide useful clues. It is normally three to six layers in thickness, depending on the state of distention. Denudation may be seen in reactive conditions (trauma or infection) or CIS. Hyperplastic urothelium may be encountered in the entire spectrum of flat intraepithelial lesions (reactive atypia, dysplasia, and CIS) and its presence mer-

TABLE 2.1. *The World Health Organization/International Society of Urological Pathology classification of flat intraurothelial lesions*

Normal
Hyperplasia
Flat lesions with atypia
    Reactive (inflammatory type)
    Dysplasia (low-grade intraurothelial lesion)
    Carcinoma in situ (high-grade intraurothelial lesion)
    Atypia of unknown significance

its evaluation of cytologic features, on the basis of which the diagnosis is ultimately made. Other features assessed at low power include polarity, nuclear crowding, and cytoplasmic clearing. In the normal urothelium, the cells are arranged perpendicularly to the basement membrane with orderly organization of the basal cells, intermediate cells, and superficial umbrella cells. Loss of normal polarity and presence of nuclear crowding are often indicative of intraurothelial neoplasia. Loss of cytoplasmic clearing (increased eosinophilia) is also a sign of dysplasia or CIS. Nucleomegaly is objectively determined by comparison if clearly normal urothelium is present in the biopsy. If normal urothelium is not present, stromal lymphocytes may also be used for size comparison. The larger nuclei in CIS are often five times the size of a normal lymphocyte, whereas the nuclear size of normal urothelium and dysplastic urothelium is only approximately twice the size of lymphocytes, aiding in their distinction from CIS (3). The presence of dysplasia is confirmed by unequivocal nuclear atypia (nuclear border and nuclear chromatin abnormalities), but does not meet the threshold for CIS. The presence of nuclear pleomorphism, frequent mitoses (including atypical mitotic figures or surface mitoses), and prominent nucleoli (single or multiple) throughout much of the urothelium favor a diagnosis of urothelial CIS over that of urothelial dysplasia or reactive changes.

TABLE 2.2. *Histologic parameters useful in the evaluation of flat lesions with atypia*

Thickness of urothelium
Polarity
Cytoplasmic clearing
Nuclear size
Nuclear crowding
Nuclear borders including notches
Nuclear chromatin distribution
Nucleoli
Mitoses including atypical forms
Accompanying inflammation
Neovascularity and inflammation at the base of
    the lesion

FEATURES OF FLAT INTRAUROTHELIAL LESION CATEGORIES

Normal

The normal urothelium, as mentioned previously, is composed of three cell types: basal, intermediate, and superficial cells arranged in three to seven cell layers, with the thickness varying depending on the state of distention (Fig. 2.1) (efigs 55–67). The basal cells are small and hyperchromatic, and they usually form a single cell layer. The intermediate cells constitute the bulk of the urothelium, the cells are oriented perpendicular to the basement membrane, and the nuclei are usually oval to round in tissue sections. Nuclear grooves are frequently identified. The cytoplasm is clear to amphophilic. The superficial or umbrella cells are arranged parallel to the basement membrane and are large, with one cell typically spanning or covering several intermediate cells (like an umbrella). The nucleus is small and cytoplasm is voluminous and clear or eosinophilic. Mild degrees of architectural variation (apparent loss of polarity) but without cytologic atypia are considered acceptable to be designated as normal (Figs. 2.2, 2.3). This is often due to tangential or thick sectioning.

SQUAMOUS METAPLASIA

Squamous metaplasia, particularly in the area of the trigone, is a common finding in women and is responsive to estrogen production (efigs 68–74). This type of squamous metaplasia is characterized by abundant intracytoplasmic glycogen and lack of keratinization, making it histologically similar to vaginal or cervical squamous epithelium (Fig. 2.4). It is likely that trigonal squamous metaplasia in women represents a normal histologic variant unassociated to local injury. Under other pathologic conditions, the metaplastic squamous epithelium undergoes keratinization and may exhibit parakeratosis and even a granular layer (4) (Fig. 2.5) (efigs 75,76). This metaplastic epithelium is not preneoplastic per

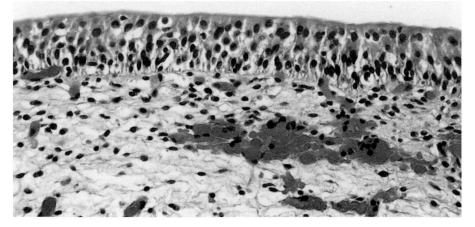

FIG. 2.1. Normal urothelium.

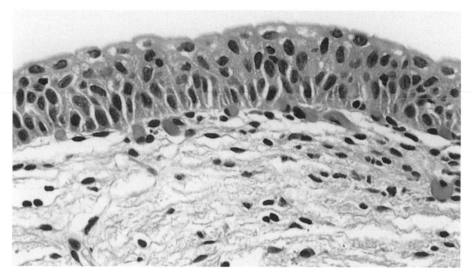

FIG. 2.2. Normal urothelium with slight disorganization and minimal variation in nuclear size and shape.

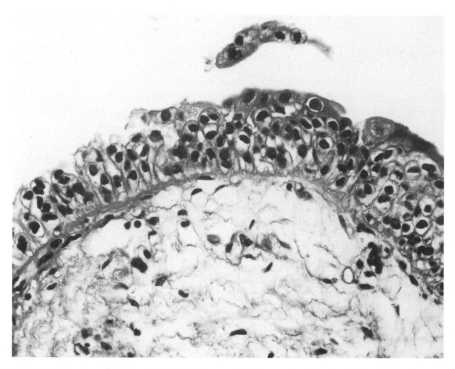

FIG. 2.3. Normal urothelium with slight disorganization and minimal variation in nuclear size and shape.

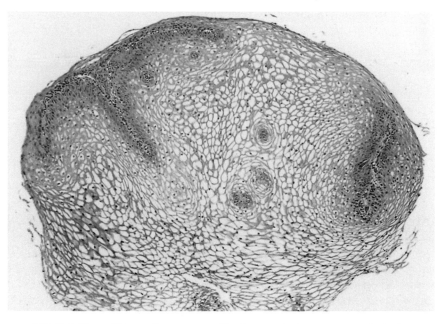

FIG. 2.4. Normal trigone in a woman with glycogenated squamous metaplasia.

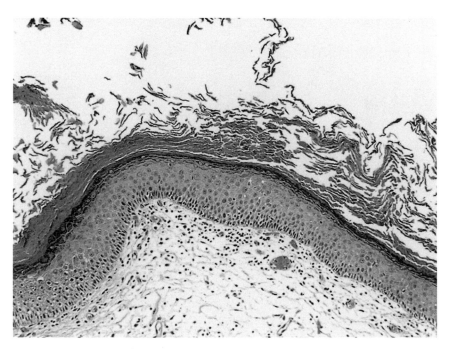

FIG. 2.5. Keratinizing squamous metaplasia.

se, but under some circumstances may lead to squamous carcinoma (see Chapter 9).

Flat Urothelial Hyperplasia

The urothelium is markedly thickened and, importantly, lacks cytologic atypia (Fig. 2.6) (efigs 77–80). Rather than requiring a specific number of cell layers, marked thickening is needed to diagnose flat hyperplasia. This lesion may be seen in the flat mucosa adjacent to low-grade papillary urothelial lesions. When seen alone, there are no data to suggest that it has a premalignant potential.

Reactive Atypia

Nucleomegaly is the most prominent finding in reactive urothelial atypia, but the cells often have a single prominent nucleolus and evenly distributed vesicular chromatin (Fig. 2.7) (efigs 81–99). The nuclei are frequently round and nuclear pleomorphism is lacking (5). Architecturally, the cells maintain their polarity perpendicular to the basement membrane. The mitotic rate may be increased with mitoses present predominantly in the basal and middle urothelium, but atypical forms are not seen. Intraurothelial acute or chronic inflamma-

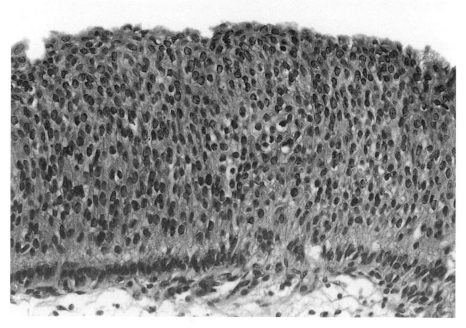

FIG. 2.6. Flat urothelial hyperplasia.

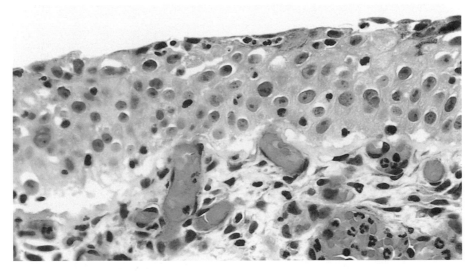

FIG. 2.7. Reactive urothelium with scattered neutrophils within urothelium.

tion is commonly identified (Figs. 2.8, 2.9). The cytoplasm may become more basophilic or eosinophilic with loss of cytoplasmic clearing. Clinical history of stones, infection, or frequent instrumentation may be present (6). Reactive urothelium may be denuded with only a single residual layer of basal cells remaining; the residual cells are not hyperchromatic, not enlarged, and do not

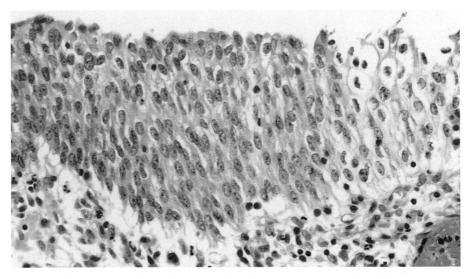

FIG. 2.8. Reactive urothelium with scattered lymphocytes and neutrophils within urothelium.

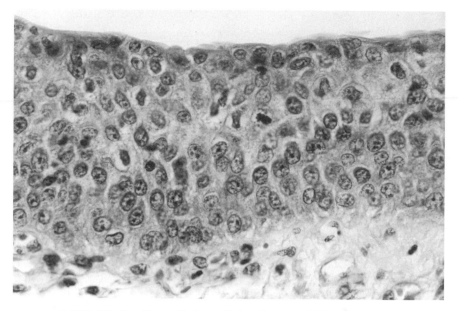

FIG. 2.9. Reactive urothelium with lymphocytes within urothelium.

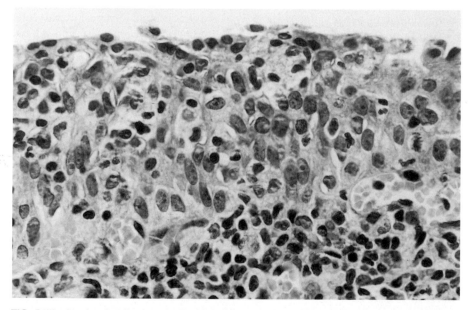

FIG. 2.10. Atypia of unknown significance with variably sized and shaped nuclei showing a mitotic figure associated with prominent inflammation that is difficult to distinguish between reactive and neoplastic atypia.

possess nuclear membrane irregularity. The umbrella cells frequently undergo reactive change alone and exhibit multinucleation or nucleomegaly, often with cytoplasmic vacuolation.

Urothelial Atypia of Unknown Significance

This term may be used as a diagnostic category in cases with inflammation in which the severity of atypia appears to be out of proportion to the extent of inflammation such that dysplasia or CIS cannot be confidently excluded (Fig. 2.10) (efigs 100,101). The message conveyed to the urologist by use of this diagnostic terminology is that the patient should be followed up after inflammation subsides. This is not a disease or diagnostic entity, but merely a descriptive term that may be designated in a biopsy in which the flat lesion with atypia cannot be diagnosed with certainty into reactive, dysplastic, or CIS categories. This term should also not be loosely used as a "wastebasket" term by pathologists for lesions with minimal atypia that may well fall into the spectrum of "normal."

Urothelial Dysplasia

Distinct appreciable nuclear abnormalities in the urothelium that occur in the absence of inflammation or that appear disproportionate to the amount of inflammation (if present), but that are not severe (i.e., falling below the threshold of CIS), may be designated as dysplasia (Figs. 2.11–2.13) (efigs 102–114). It has been proposed that bladder intraepithelial lesions, like intraepithelial lesions of the cervix, be graded on the basis of level of involvement of atypical cells (i.e., mild dysplasia for lesions showing atypia confined to the lower one third, moderate dysplasia for atypia up to the middle third, and so on) (7). However, observations in animal models and in clinical specimens indicate that atypia progresses quantitatively and qualitatively from dysplasia to CIS, stressing the importance of cytologic features rather than histologic pattern (i.e., on the level of atypia) (8).

In dysplasia, the thickness of the urothelium is usually normal (four to seven layers) but may be increased or decreased. Flat lesions with a benign cytology and minimal disorder should be considered within the spectrum of "normal" (1). Dysplastic lesions show loss of polarity (normal cells are columnar to oval with nuclei perpendicular to the basement membrane) evidenced by crowding and more rounded to polygonal cells with nuclei parallel to the long axis. Nuclear atypia is evident but is not severe enough to merit a diagnosis of CIS. Often, increased cytoplasmic eosinophilia, nucleomegaly, irregularity of nuclear contours with notching of cell borders, and altered chromatin distribution are seen. Nucleoli are usually not conspicuous; only a minimal degree of pleomorphism is allowable in dysplasia, and the mitotic activity is variable although usually not in the higher layers. The lamina propria is usually unaltered, but it may contain increased inflammation or neovascularity. Denudation with atypical cells cling-

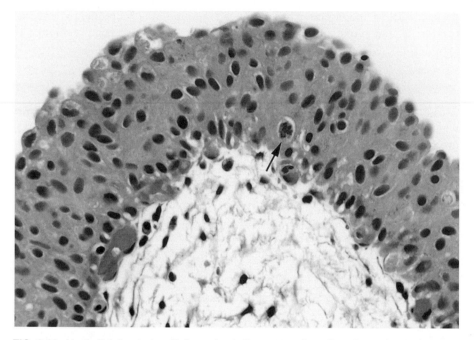

FIG. 2.11. Urothelial dysplasia with loss of polarity, scattered small yet hyperchromatic nuclei, and a mitotic figure (*arrow*).

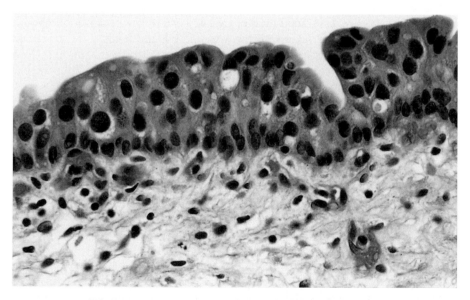

FIG. 2.12. Urothelial dysplasia with scattered, enlarged nuclei.

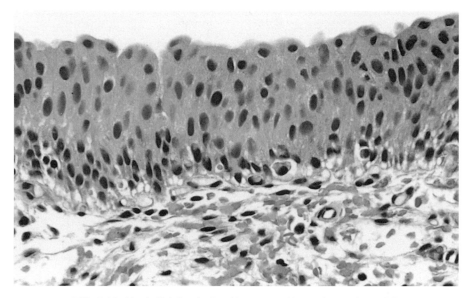

FIG. 2.13. Urothelial dysplasia with scattered hyperchromatic nuclei.

ing to the submucosa is not a common feature of dysplasia. Comparison with more normal appearing urothelium, if present in the same biopsy specimen or in another simultaneously obtained biopsy specimen from the same patient, may help in assessing features such as nucleomegaly, loss of clearing, and loss of polarity. A diagnosis of primary dysplasia (i.e., no prior history or concomitant urothelial neoplasia) should be made with great caution.

Dysplasia is usually a histologic diagnosis seen most commonly in patients with bladder neoplasia, in whom the incidence is 22% to 86%. The incidence approaches 100% in patients with invasive carcinoma. Little is known about de novo dysplasia because there is a lack of screening in the general population. Furthermore, de novo dysplasia is usually cystoscopically and clinically silent, although it may appear as a slightly raised and mildly erythematous patch. The patients are predominantly middle-aged men presenting occasionally with irritative bladder symptoms with or without hematuria. The few studies published on de novo dysplasia indicate that 5% to 19% of patients progress to have urothelial neoplasia (9–12). The finding of dysplasia in patients with bladder cancer suggests that it is a marker for progression (increased recurrences or future invasion) (13–15). The definition of dysplasia used in these studies has been variable, so their true clinical meaning remains in doubt.

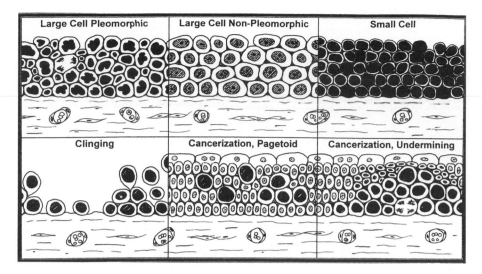

FIG. 2.14. Schematic representations of carcinoma in situ. (From McKenney JK, Gomez JA, Desai S, et al. Morphologic expressions of urothelial carcinoma in situ: a detailed evaluation of its histologic patterns with emphasis on carcinoma in situ with microinvasion. *Am J Surg Pathol* 2001;25:356–362, with permission.)

Urothelial Carcinoma In Situ

Unequivocal severe cytologic atypia (i.e., changes thought to represent clear-cut neoplasia at the light microscopic level) is necessary for the diagnosis of CIS (Color Plate 1) (efigs 115–173). The urothelium may be denuded, reflecting the discohesive nature of the cells; it may be diminished in thickness, be of normal thickness, or even be hyperplastic. Denudation, however, may be produced artifactually by the biopsy procedure, especially if the biopsy is performed with a hot wire loop (16). There may be alteration or complete loss of polarity, marked crowding, pleomorphism, and frequent mitoses. The lamina propria is frequently hypervascular and inflamed, reflecting the erythematous appearance witnessed on cystoscopy. The nuclear anaplasia is generally obvious, although a spectrum

TABLE 2.3. *Histologic patterns of urothelial carcinoma in situ[a]*

Large cell, pleomorphic
Large cell, nonpleomorphic
Small cell
Clinging
Cancerization of normal urothelium
    Pagetoid
    Undermining/Overriding

[a]It is important for pathologists to recognize the different histologic patterns of carcinoma in situ; however, they need not be subclassified in the pathology report because individual patterns do not carry any known clinical significance.

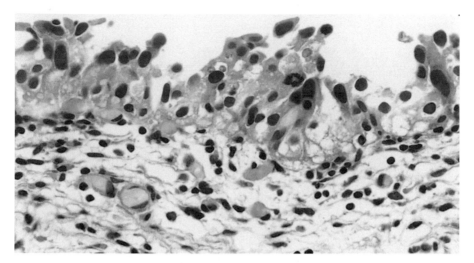

FIG. 2.15. Carcinoma in situ.

of severity may exist. Additionally, there are varied cytologic and architectural patterns in the histologic presentation of CIS (17,18) (Fig. 2.14) (Table 2.3).

The pattern of CIS that is most easily recognized is large cell CIS with pleomorphism (Figs. 2.15–2.17). The neoplastic cells show considerable loss of polarity and nucleomegaly with marked variation in nuclear shape and size, but

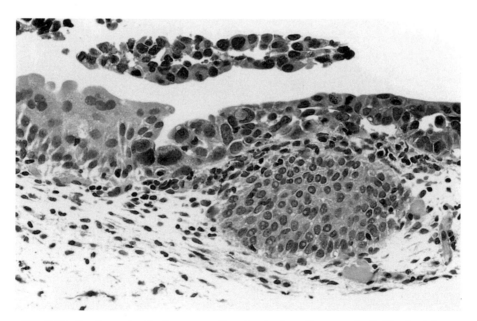

FIG. 2.16. Carcinoma in situ. Compare with uninvolved von Brunn nest with bland cytology.

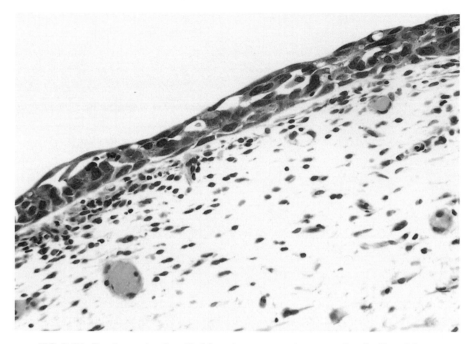

FIG. 2.17. Carcinoma in situ with thinned mucosa and preserved umbrella cell layer.

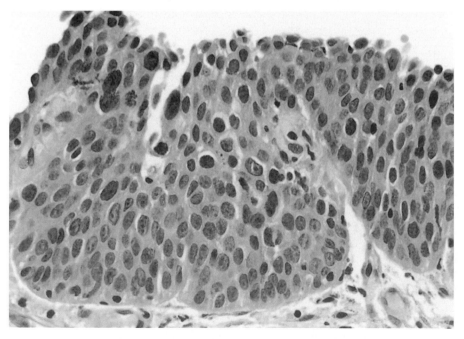

FIG. 2.18. Carcinoma in situ with prominent nucleoli.

retain abundant eosinophilic cytoplasm. The neoplastic cells in other examples of CIS may be monomorphic (large cell CIS without pleomorphism) (Fig. 2.18). These lesions may mimic reactive urothelial atypia because of the uniformity of the cells with conspicuous eosinophilic cytoplasm; however, they have markedly enlarged nuclei with high-grade cytologic features diagnostic of CIS. Small cell CIS has nuclear features identical to large cell CIS without pleomorphism, but it has scant cytoplasm (Fig. 2.19). There is no precursor relationship to small cell carcinoma of the bladder or any neuroendocrine connotation; this is merely a descriptive designation. Although the cells appear smaller because of the absence of significant cytoplasm, the nuclei are still markedly enlarged with nuclear chromatin abnormalities. CIS cells tend to be discohesive, wherein they can be seen lifting off the basement membrane (Figs. 2.20, 2.21). Clinging CIS is characterized by a partially denuded urothelium with a patchy, usually single layer of residual urothelial cells meeting the morphologic criteria for CIS (Figs. 2.22, 2.23) (efigs 136–139).

CIS may also show cancerization of normal urothelium in two patterns: (a) pagetoid spread with the presence of clusters or isolated single cells with features of CIS within normal urothelium and (b) undermining or overriding of the normal urothelium by adjacent CIS of any other pattern (Figs. 2.24–2.26) (efigs 146–156). Rare cases of CIS may also show glandlike differentiation. In routine diagnostic practice, we report all CIS cases as simply "urothelial carcinoma in situ" and do not include a descriptor of the particular pattern of CIS in the line diagnosis. The terms *large cell nonpleomorphic* and *clinging* help pathologists recognize the important lesion of CIS, especially because there is a wide range in its morphologic presentation. The prognostic implications of the different pat-

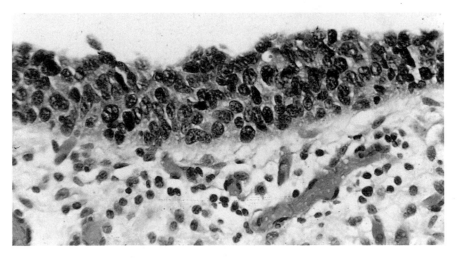

FIG. 2.19. Small cell urothelial carcinoma in situ.

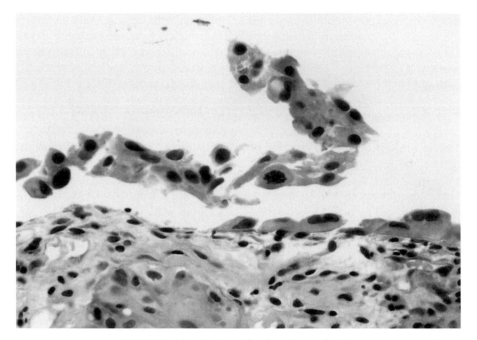

FIG. 2.20. Discohesive cells of carcinoma in situ.

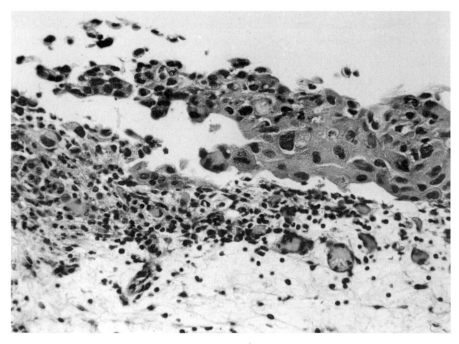

FIG. 2.21. Discohesive cells of carcinoma in situ.

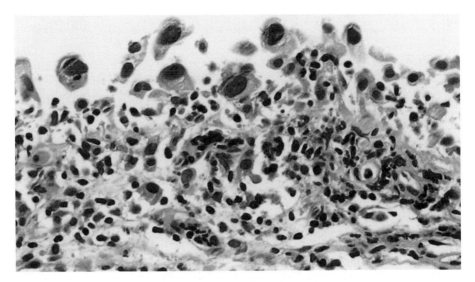

FIG. 2.22. Clinging carcinoma in situ.

terns of CIS are not known, and the use of descriptors of CIS, such as clinging or pagetoid, in the surgical pathology report could potentially lead to confusion on the part of the treating urologist. CIS must also be distinguished from squamous cell CIS (see Chapter 9) (efigs 174–177).

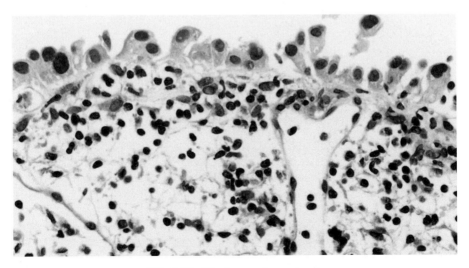

FIG. 2.23. Clinging carcinoma in situ.

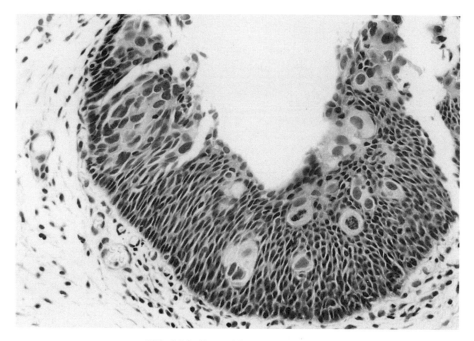

FIG. 2.24. Pagetoid carcinoma in situ.

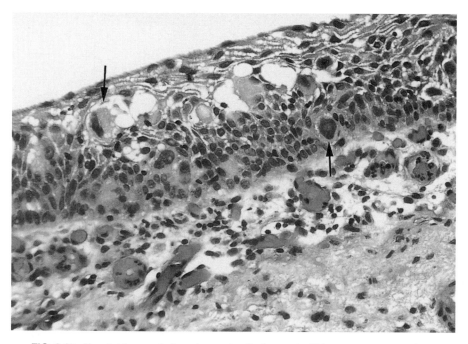

FIG. 2.25. Pagetoid spread of carcinoma in situ (*arrows*) within squamous metaplasia.

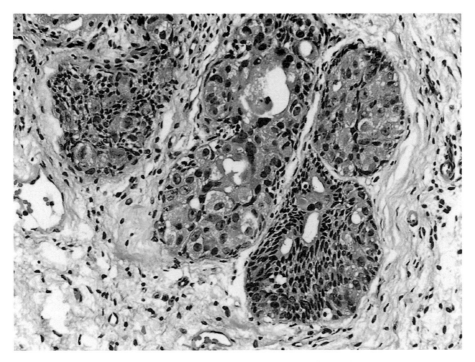

FIG. 2.26. Pagetoid spread of carcinoma in situ within von Brunn nests.

Distinction of dysplasia from CIS is one morphologic threshold (efigs 168–173). The presence of full thickness nuclear atypia, pleomorphism, prominent nucleoli throughout the urothelium, or mitoses in the upper urothelium, particularly atypical forms, favors the diagnosis of CIS over dysplasia.

Distinction of CIS from reactive conditions can be difficult, although in most instances it is straightforward based on nuclear characteristics. In the experience of one of the authors (M.B.A.), a panel of immunohistochemical antibodies consisting of cytokeratin 20 (CK20), p53, and CD44 (standard isoform) may have utility in the distinction of CIS from reactive atypia (5,19,20). A panel consisting of these three antibodies is important because not all cases of CIS consistently exhibit the characteristic immunostaining specified in the subsequent discussion. Normal urothelium shows reactivity for CK20 only in the superficial umbrella cell layer, whereas CD44 staining is limited to the basal and parabasal urothelial cells. Nuclear staining for p53 is absent to focal in normal urothelium. Urothelium with reactive atypia shows increased reactivity for CD44 in all layers of the urothelium, particularly in cases with marked atypia. In reactive urothelium, CK20 and p53 reactivity patterns are usually identical to those seen in normal urothelium. In contrast, CIS frequently shows diffuse, strong cytoplasmic reactivity for CK20 and diffuse nuclear reactivity for p53 throughout the full thickness of the urothelium. CD44 reactivity is limited to a residual basal cell layer of normal urothelium when present, but is often absent in the neoplastic cells. These findings are based on immunohistochemical correlation in morphologically unequivocal cases of CIS and reactive atypia, performed retrospectively. This panel is potentially useful as an adjunct to morphology in several diagnostic situations: (a) in cases in which the pathologist strongly favors the diagnosis of CIS but has reservations making a definitive diagnosis; (b) in the diagnosis of CIS at initial presentation with no known history of a papillary lesion (de novo or primary CIS); and (c) in confirming unusual morphologic presentations of CIS such as the cancerization of normal urothelium.

The clinical course and biologic potential of CIS is better understood chiefly because it is more often symptomatic and may be detected by cystoscopy, rendering it recognizable in a primary or de novo form. Most patients present with frequency, dysuria, nocturia, and suprapubic fullness; hematuria is typically microscopic (21,22). The bladder at cystoscopy appears erythematous or granular, although no abnormality may be present. The biologic potential of CIS is somewhat unpredictable, although the current dogma states that it is a precursor to invasive carcinoma. The aggregate evidence in the literature suggests that invasive carcinoma will develop in up to one half of the patients within 5 years (15). From a clinical perspective, extent of disease (focal, multifocal, or extensive), involvement of prostatic urethra, and response to therapy are the principal determinants of clinical outcome. Patients with primary (de novo) CIS are more likely to have no evidence of disease (62% versus 45%) and are less likely to progress (28% versus 59%) or die of disease (7% versus 45%) when compared with patients with CIS occurring in patients with papillary bladder neoplasia (23).

PROBLEMS AND PITFALLS IN THE DIAGNOSIS OF FLAT LESIONS WITH ATYPIA

Innate Vagaries of Normal Urothelium and Histologic Sectioning

The thickness of the normal urothelium varies with the state of distention of the bladder. If the sections are thick, the urothelium may appear hyperchromatic, and this artifact, compounded with tangential sectioning, may result in changes thought to represent dysplasia. The urothelium of the renal pelvis, urethra, and bladder neck is usually composed of cells with slightly larger nuclei and diminished cytoplasmic clearing and, hence, may be misinterpreted as dysplasia.

Inflammatory Atypia

The presence of acute or significant chronic inflammation, particularly in an intraurothelial location, warrants caution in the interpretation of dysplasia or CIS, although inflammatory atypia may coexist with dysplasia or CIS.

Therapy-Associated Atypia

Upon cursory examination, these changes could easily be mistaken for intraepithelial neoplasia. Radiation can induce full thickness atypia closely mimicking CIS; however, there are often multinucleated cells with bizarre nuclei not typical of intraurothelial neoplasia (see Chapter 10). The cytoplasm in radiation atypia is often prominent and may show degenerative changes with vacuolization. Other associated changes may be identified in the bladder wall, including atypical fibroblasts and radiation vasculopathy. Intravesical chemotherapy can also induce severe urothelial atypia, but it is usually more prominent in the superficial urothelial cells.

Extensive Denudation

Trauma due to instrumentation, prior therapy, and CIS are the main conditions associated with denudation. The presence of a few atypical single cells clinging to the surface is sometimes the only sign of CIS ("denuding cystitis"); deeper sections through the block may reveal diagnostic cells. In the absence of atypical cells, the finding of extensive denudation, particularly that associated with neovascularity and chronic inflammation in the lamina propria, must be included in the report, and correlation with urine cytology findings may be suggested. In cases of true denuding cystitis resulting from CIS, urine or bladder wash cytology may contain a large number of neoplastic cells.

Truncated Papillae of Treated Papillary Carcinoma

Mitomycin C and thiotepa therapy destroys the tips of the papillae of papillary urothelial carcinoma because they act as surface abrasives. When these truncated papillae are seen in areas associated with denudation and inflammation, they may be mistaken for CIS or dysplastic changes instead of residual papillary urothelial carcinoma (Fig. 2.27) (24). An unusual form of CIS that could mimic truncated papillae of treated papillary carcinoma is CIS with micropapillary features (Fig. 2.28) (efig 178–179).

Carcinoma In Situ Involving von Brunn Nests: Overdiagnosis of Invasion

CIS can involve von Brunn nests, resulting in the presence of neoplastic cells within the superficial lamina propria (Fig. 2.29). In general, von Brunn nests have a round contour and lack retraction artifact or surrounding stromal changes. In the presence of inflammation, however, the basement membrane may be obscured and distorted, simulating invasion.

Carcinoma In Situ with Microinvasion: Underdiagnosis of Invasion

A histologically subtle, but potentially ominous, clinical situation arises when CIS is associated with microinvasion (see Chapter 5). The urologist is most often

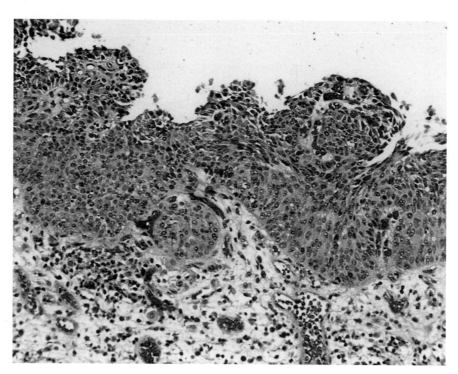

FIG. 2.27. Truncated papillae in papillary urothelial carcinoma following intravesical chemotherapy.

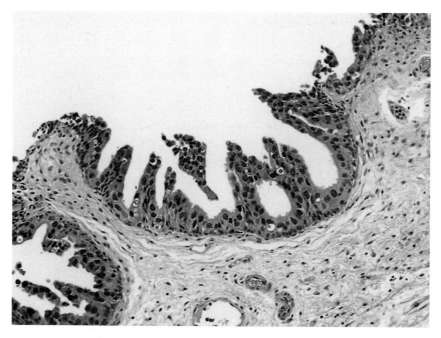

FIG. 2.28. Carcinoma in situ with micropapillary features.

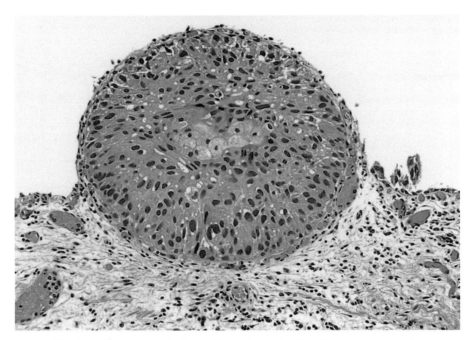

FIG. 2.29. Denuded urothelium with carcinoma in situ within von Brunn nests.

unsuspecting of invasive disease on the basis of cystoscopic evaluation, and the pathologist may fail to recognize single cell invasion or small clusters of invasion that may be camouflaged by background inflammation. Desmoplasia or retraction artifact is useful in recognizing invasion, but a stromal response may be absent (5,25).

Polyomavirus Infection

Infection of immunocompromised patients with the human polyomavirus, usually a nonpathogenic virus, results in large homogeneous inclusions in enlarged nuclei of urothelial cells, or "decoy cells" (see Chapter 10). The findings are more frequently seen in urine cytology but may rarely be found on biopsy; in both specimens, malignancy (CIS) is mimicked (26).

REFERENCES

1. Epstein JI, Amin MB, Reuter VE, et al. The World Health Organization/International Society of Urological Pathology consensus classification of urothelial (transitional cell) neoplasms of the urinary bladder. *Am J Surg Pathol* 1998;22:1435–1448.
2. Amin MB, McKenney JK. An approach to the diagnosis of flat intraepithelial lesions of the urinary bladder using the World Health Organization/International Society of Urological Pathology (WHO/ISUP) consensus classification system. *Adv Anat Pathol* 2002;9:222–232.

3. Milford RA, Lecksell K, Epstein JI. An objective morphologic parameter to aid in the diagnosis of flat urothelial carcinoma in situ. *Hum Pathol* 2001;32:997–1002.
4. Tannenbaum M. Inflammatory proliferative lesion of the urinary bladder: squamous metaplasia. *Urology* 1976;7:428–429.
5. McKenney JK, Desai S, Cohen C, et al. Discriminatory immunohistochemical staining of urothelial carcinoma in situ and non-neoplastic urothelium. An analysis of cytokeratin 20, p53, and CD44 antigens. *Am J Surg Pathol* 2001;25:1074–1078.
6. Amin MB, Young RH. Intraepithelial lesions of the urinary bladder with a discussion of the histogenesis of urothelial neoplasia. *Semin Diag Pathol* 1997;14:84–97.
7. Ayala AG, Ro JY. Premalignant lesions of urothelium and transitional cell tumors. In: Young RH, ed. *Contemporary issues in surgical pathology: pathology of the urinary bladder*. New York: Churchill Livingstone, 1989:65–101.
8. Murphy WM, Soloway MS. Developing carcinoma (dysplasia) of the urinary bladder. In: Sommers SC, Rosen PP, eds. *Pathology annual*, 17. Norwalk, CT: Appleton-Century-Crofts, 1982:197–217.
9. Zuk RJ, Rogers HS, Martin JE, et al. Clinicopathological importance of primary dysplasia of bladder. *J Clin Pathol* 1988;41:1277–1280.
10. Murphy WM, Miller AW. In: Javadpour NE, ed. *Bladder cancer*. Baltimore: Williams & Wilkins, 1984:100–122.
11. Smith G, Elton RA, Beynon LL. Prognostic significance of biopsy results of normal-looking mucosa in cases of superficial bladder cancer. *Br J Urol* 1983;55:665–669.
12. Althausen AF, Prout GRJ, Dal JJ. Noninvasive papillary carcinoma of the bladder associated with carcinoma-in-situ. *J Urol* 1976;116:575–580.
13. Mostofi FK, Sesterhenn IA. Pathology of epithelial tumors and carcinoma in situ of bladder: bladder cancer: A. *Prog Clin Biol Res* 1984;162A:55–74.
14. Cheng L, Cheville JC, Neumann RM, et al. Natural history of urothelial dysplasia of the bladder. *Am J Surg Pathol* 1999;23:443–447.
15. Cheng L, Cheville JC, Neumann RM, et al. Flat intraurothelial lesions of the urinary bladder. *Cancer* 2000;88:625–631.
16. Levi AW, Potter SR, Schoenberg MP, et al. Clinical significance of denuded urothelium in bladder biopsy. *J Urol* 2001;166:457–460.
17. Amin MB, Murphy WM, Reuter VE, et al. Controversies in the pathology of transitional cell carcinoma of the urinary bladder. In Rosen PP, Fechner RE, eds. *Reviews in pathology*, Chicago: ASCP Press, 1996:1–38.
18. McKenney JK, Gomez JA, Desai S, et al. Morphologic expressions of urothelial carcinoma in situ: a detailed evaluation of its histologic patterns with emphasis on carcinoma in situ with microinvasion. *Am J Surg Pathol* 2001;25:356–362.
19. Sarkis AS, Dalbagni G, Cordon-Cardo C, et al. Association of p53 nuclear overexpression and tumor progression in carcinoma in situ of the bladder. *J Urol* 1994;152:388–392.
20. Harnden P, Eardley I, Joyce AD, et al. Cytokeratin 20 as an objective marker of urothelial dysplasia. *Br J Urol* 1996;78:870–875.
21. Lamm DL. Carcinoma in situ. *Urol Clin North Am* 1992;19:499–508.
22. Murphy WM, Soloway MS. Urothelial dysplasia. *J Urol* 1982;127:849–854.
23. Orozco RE, Martin AA, Murphy WM. Carcinoma in situ of the urinary bladder: clues to host involvement in human carcinogenesis. *Cancer* 1994;76:115–122.
24. Murphy WM, Soloway MS, Finebaum PJ. Pathologic changes associated with topical chemotherapy for superficial bladder cancer. *J Urol* 1980;126:461–465.
25. Amin MB, Gomez JA, Young RH. Urothelial transitional cell carcinoma with endophytic growth patterns. A discussion of patterns of invasion and problems associated with carcinoma-in-situ. *Am J Surg Pathol* 1997;21:1057–1068.
26. Koss LG. *Diagnostic cytology and its histopathologic basis*, 4th ed. Philadelphia: JB Lippincott, 1992.

3

Papillary Urothelial Neoplasms and Their Precursors

The World Health Organization (WHO)/International Society of Urological Pathologists (ISUP) classification of noninvasive papillary urothelial lesions is outlined in Table 3.1 (1). The diagnosis of lesions within this classification takes into account architectural and cytologic features within the urothelium (Table 3.2).

PAPILLARY UROTHELIAL HYPERPLASIA

At least one study suggests that papillary urothelial hyperplasia is a likely precursor lesion to low-grade papillary urothelial neoplasms. Typically they are discovered on routine follow-up cystoscopy for papillary urothelial neoplasms and less frequently in the workup for microhematuria or urinary obstructive symptoms. In most cases at cystoscopy, a focal elevated lesion is identified that is variably described as "bleblike," "papillary," "raised," "sessile," or "frondular" (2).

Histologically, papillary hyperplasia consists of undulating urothelium arranged into mucosal narrow papillary folds of varying heights (Fig. 3.1) (efigs 180–190). Both the urothelium within papillary hyperplasia and the adjacent flat mucosa are often thicker than normal. In addition to the diagnostic mucosal folds, in some cases there are also tent-shaped, somewhat broader folds that lack the edema and inflammation typical of polypoid cystitis. The cytologic findings in typical papillary hyperplasia are similar to that in normal urothelium. Some cases show increased vascularity in the stroma at the base of the papillary folds. An occasional case may also demonstrate early slight branching beginning at the top of one of the folds of papillary hyperplasia. Papillary hyperplasia is distinguished from papillary urothelial neoplasms by a lack of arborization and absence of "detached" papillary fronds (Fig. 3.2).

Large studies with sufficient follow-up to evaluate the clinical significance of de novo papillary hyperplasia are lacking. Nevertheless, even though de novo

TABLE 3.1. *The World Health Organization/International Society of Urological Pathology consensus classification of papillary urothelial (transitional cell) lesions*

Hyperplasia
    Papillary hyperplasia
Papillary neoplasms
    Papilloma
    Papillary neoplasm of low malignant potential
    Papillary carcinoma, low-grade
    Papillary carcinoma, high-grade

papillary hyperplasia will not inevitably progress to urothelial neoplasia, it is reasonable to suggest that patients should be followed up more closely than persons in the general population. If papillary hyperplasia is diagnosed in someone with a history of urothelial neoplasia, it most likely indicates early recurrence of papillary neoplasia and warrants continued close follow-up.

TABLE 3.2. *Histologic features of papillary urothelial lesions*

	Papilloma	Papillary neoplasm of low malignant potential	Low-grade papillary carcinoma	High-grade papillary carcinoma
Architecture				
Papillae	Delicate	Delicate; occasionally fused	Fused; branching; delicate	Fused; branching; delicate
Organization of cells	Identical to normal	Polarity identical to normal; any thickness; cohesive	Predominantly ordered, yet minimal crowding and minimal loss of polarity; any thickness; cohesive	Predominantly disordered with frequent loss of polarity; any thickness; often discohesive
Cytology				
Nuclear size	Identical to normal	May be uniformly enlarged	Enlarged with variation in size	Enlarged with variation in size
Nuclear shape	Identical to normal	Elongated; round–oval; uniform	Round–oval; slight variation in shape and contour	Moderate–marked pleomorphism
Nuclear chromatin	Fine	Fine	Mild variation within and between cells	Moderate–marked variation within and between cells with hyperchromasia
Nucleoli	Absent	Absent to inconspicuous	Usually inconspicuous[a]	Multiple prominent nucleoli may be present
Mitoses	Absent	Rare; basal	Occasional, at any level	Usually frequent, at any level; may be atypical
Umbrella cells	Uniformly present	Present	Usually present	May be present

[a]If present, small and regular and not accompanied by other features of high-grade carcinoma.

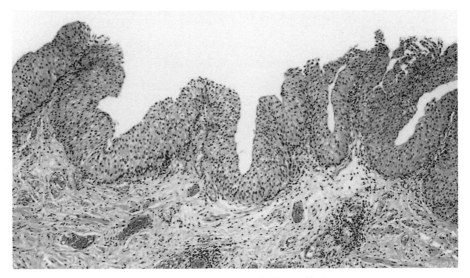

FIG. 3.1. Papillary urothelial hyperplasia.

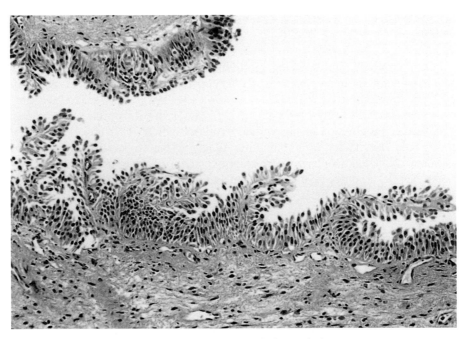

FIG. 3.2. Papillary urothelial hyperplasia.

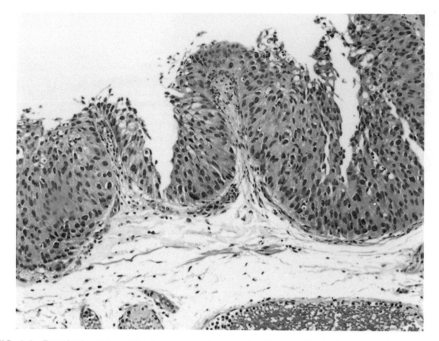

FIG. 3.3. Dysplasia with architecture of papillary urothelial hyperplasia (some would regard as low-grade papillary urothelial cancer).

Less commonly, the overlying urothelium in a lesion with the architectural pattern of papillary hyperplasia reveals varying degrees of cytologic atypia ranging from dysplasia to CIS (3) (Fig. 3.3) (efigs 191–193). One hypothesis is that, in some cases, CIS or dysplasia may evolve into atypical papillary hyperplasia, with further progression to high-grade papillary cancer. This process is analogous to papillary hyperplasia without cytologic atypia progressing to low-grade papillary urothelial neoplasms. The other explanation is that these represent urethelial neoplasia somewhere between flat and papillary disease and, if the patient had received prior treatment, could be an effect of therapy.

PAPILLARY UROTHELIAL NEOPLASMS

Background

The classification and grading of papillary urothelial neoplasms has been a long-standing source of controversy (4). There are numerous grading systems, most of which have poor interobserver reproducibility, with most cases falling into an intermediate category (5–12). The most commonly used grading systems for bladder tumors have been those proposed by WHO. In 1973, the WHO system proposed that tumors be categorized into benign urothelial papillomas and three grades of carcinoma (grades 1, 2, and 3) (13). A major limitation of the WHO (1973) grading system was its vague definition of the various grades and its lack of specific histologic criteria. The following statement is the sole description of the difference between WHO grades 1, 2, and 3 as written in the original WHO (1973) system: "Grade 1 tumors have the least degree of anaplasia compatible with the diagnosis of malignancy. Grade 3 applies to tumors with the most severe degrees of cellular anaplasia, and Grade 2 lies in between" (7). In December 1998, members of WHO and ISUP published the WHO/ISUP consensus classification of urothelial (transitional cell) neoplasms of the urinary bladder (1). This new classification system arose out of the need to develop a more detailed classification system for bladder neoplasia and because many of the tumors classified as "transitional cell carcinoma, grade 1" had no potential for malignant behavior once completely excised. In 1999, the WHO revised its classification system in response to the WHO/ISUP system. This revision retains most of the WHO/ISUP system, yet differs in one key respect, which is all the more perplexing in that one of the leading members of the 1999 WHO system was also an author on the WHO/ISUP system. Furthermore, grades 1, 2, and 3 in the 1973 WHO system are not the same as grades 1, 2, 3 in the 1999 WHO system (see below). In 2003, WHO revised its classification of urothelial tumors, adopting the WHO/ISUP system in its original version, resulting in a unified grading system for urothelial tumors (13). Because these systems are identical, in this text, the grading system is referred to as the WHO(2003)/ISUP system.

WHO(2003)/ISUP System

The WHO(2003)/ISUP system is a modified version of the scheme proposed by Malmström and colleagues (10). One of the major contributions of the WHO(2003)/ISUP system is a detailed histologic description of the various grades, using specific cytologic and architectural criteria. These criteria are based on the architectural features relating to the histology of the papillae and the overall organization of the cells. Cytologic features encompassed in the WHO(2003)/ISUP system include nuclear size, nuclear shape, chromatin content, nucleoli, mitoses, and umbrella cells. Papillary tumors may show heterogeneity of grade. Tumors are graded based on the highest grade exhibited, although it remains to be defined what percentage is minimally needed to place tumors in a higher category when the highest grade is focal. The terminology used in the WHO(2003)/ISUP system is somewhat consistent with that used in urine cytology. Having a consensus classification between cytology and histopathology is also advantageous. To further improve the accuracy with which the WHO(2003)/ISUP system is used, a website has been developed that illustrates numerous examples of the various grades: *www.pathology.jhu.edu/bladder*.

Relation of WHO (1973) to WHO(2003)/ISUP

A major misconception in the application of the WHO(2003)/ISUP classification is that there is a one-to-one translation between it and the WHO (1973) classification system (Fig. 3.4). Only at the extremes of grades in the WHO

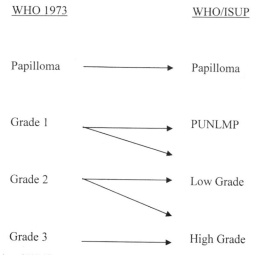

FIG. 3.4. Relationship of WHO 1973 to WHO(2003)/ISUP classification of papillary urothelial tumors.

(1973) classification does this one-to-one correlation hold true. Lesions called papilloma in the WHO (1973) classification system are also called papilloma in the WHO(2003)/ISUP system. At the other end of the grading extreme, lesions called WHO (1973) grade 3 are by definition high-grade carcinoma in the WHO(2003)/ISUP system. However, for WHO (1973) grades 1 and 2, there is no direct translation to WHO(2003)/ISUP classification system. Rather, lesions must be analyzed using the criteria of the WHO(2003)/ISUP classification system without regard to how they were diagnosed in WHO (1973) system. Lesions formerly called WHO (1973) grade 1, which upon review show no cytologic atypia and merely thickened urothelium with, at most, nuclear enlargement, would be called papillary urothelial neoplasms of low malignant potential (PUNLMP). However, other WHO (1973) grade 1 lesions with definite yet slight cytologic atypia, would be diagnosed in the WHO (2003)/ISUP system as low-grade urothelial carcinomas. Within the WHO (1973) system, grade 2 is a very broad category. It includes lesions that are relatively bland, which in some places are diagnosed as WHO (1973) grade 1-2; these lesions in the WHO(2003)/ISUP system would be called papillary urothelial low-grade carcinoma. In other cases, WHO (1973) grade 2 lesions border on higher grade lesions and, in many institutions, are called WHO (1973) grade 2-3; these lesions in the WHO (2003)/ISUP classification system would be called high-grade carcinoma.

Papilloma

Using the WHO (1973) system, some experts applied very restrictive criteria for the diagnosis of urothelial papilloma, in part based on the number of cell layers, and regarded all other papillary neoplasms as carcinomas. Others applied a broader definition of "urothelial papilloma" so as not to label all patients with papillary lesions with minimal cytologic and architectural atypia as having carcinoma.

The WHO(2003)/ISUP system has very restrictive histologic features for the diagnosis of papilloma, requiring papillary fronds to be lined by normal appearing urothelium (Figs. 3.5–3.11) (efigs 194–237). Most papillomas present as single lesions that are relatively small. However, multifocal tumors and larger lesions may be seen.

Most papillomas have a simple nonbranching or minimally branching arrangement, slender fibrovascular stalks, and a predominantly exophytic pattern. In some papillomas, more complex anastomosing papillae, marked stromal edema within the papillae, and endophytic areas (areas of inverted papilloma (efig 238) can be identified (Figs. 3.12, 3.13).

Within the limits of normal urothelial thickness, there is some variability. Uncommon cases may be composed of only one to two cell layers of urothelium. There is no need to count the maximum number of cell layers, as long as it not obviously thicker than the normal urothelial lining. In most cases, the urothelium is tightly cohesive, although in some cases there may be the appearance of dis-

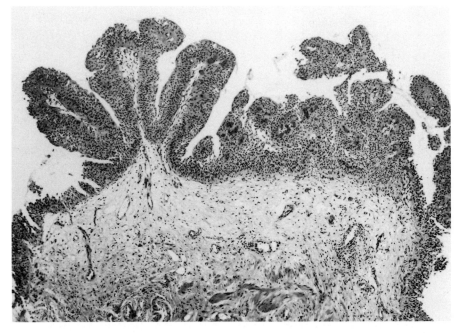

FIG. 3.5. Early papilloma with branching of papillae (left) with more well-developed small papillary fronds (right).

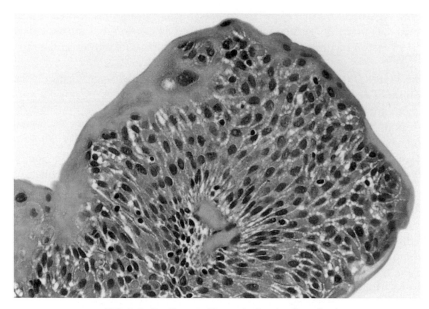

FIG. 3.6. Papilloma with atypical umbrella cells.

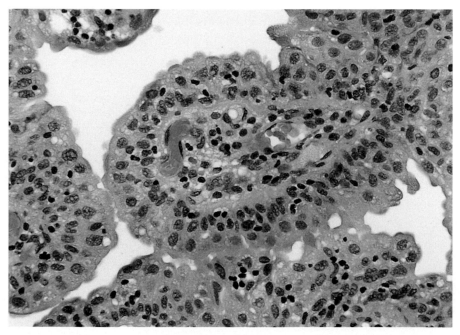

FIG. 3.7. Papilloma.

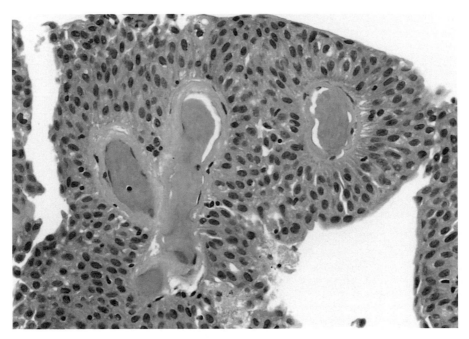

FIG. 3.8. Papilloma.

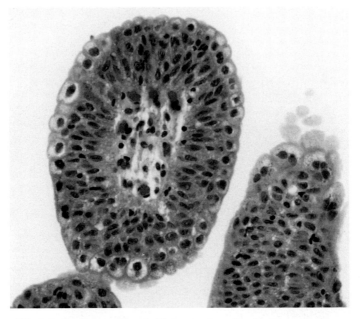

FIG. 3.9. Papilloma with cuboidal umbrella cells with clear cytoplasm.

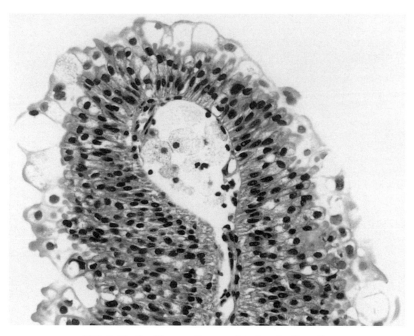

FIG. 3.10. Papilloma with vacuolated umbrella cells.

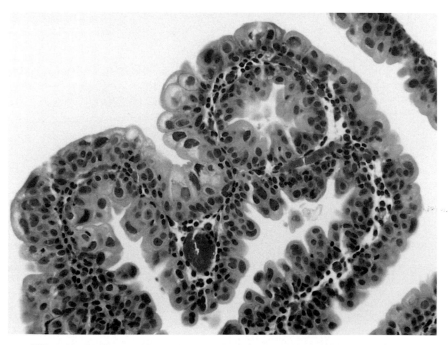

FIG. 3.11. Papilloma with prominent umbrella cells showing hobnail morphology.

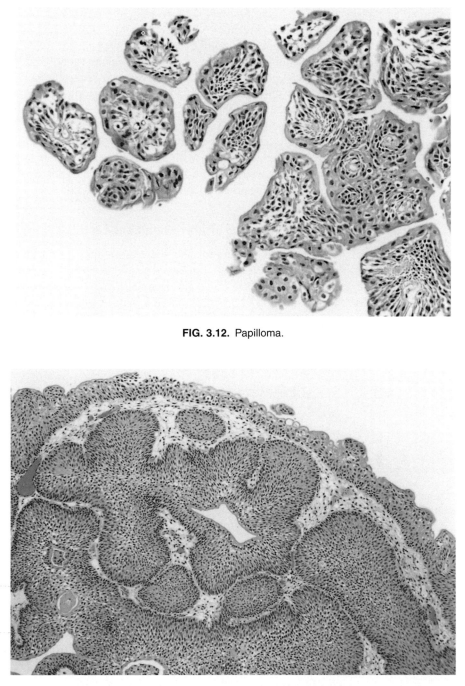

FIG. 3.12. Papilloma.

FIG. 3.13. Areas of the tumor seen in Figure 3.12 showed inverted papilloma consistent with mixed exophytic and inverted urothelial papilloma.

cohesion. Umbrella cells vary in their morphology from being inconspicuous, to being cuboidal with slightly enlarged nuclei and paler cytoplasm, to having a hobnail appearance with abundant eosinophilic cytoplasm. Occasional cases of urothelial papilloma have an umbrella cell layer with prominent vacuolization. Single, enlarged umbrella cells may also drape themselves over several underlying urothelial cells, where the umbrella cell nuclei may demonstrate degenerative atypia. Urothelial atypia, other than that which can be seen in umbrella cells, excludes the diagnosis of papilloma.

Papillomas are rare and typically, but not exclusinvely, occur in younger patients. Papillomas may occur in association with a prior or concurrent history of other urothelial tumors. However, if a papilloma is the first manifestation of urothelial neoplasia, most of these lesions, once resected, do not recur (14).

Papillary Urothelial Neoplasm of Low Malignant Potential

The category of PUNLMP was derived to describe lesions that do not have cytologic features of malignancy, yet have thickened urothelium as compared with papilloma (Figs. 3.14–3.19) (Color Plate 2) (efigs 239–276). Having a category of PUNLMP avoids labeling a patient as having cancer, which has psychosocial and financial (e.g., insurance) implications, but neither is a benign

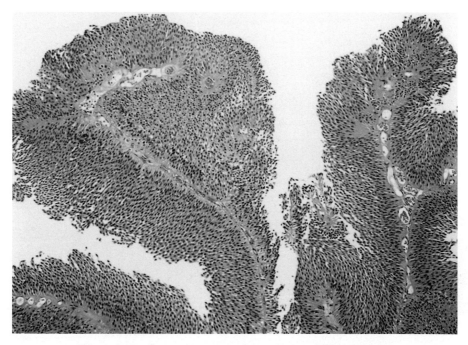

FIG. 3.14. Papillary urothelial neoplasm of low malignant potential.

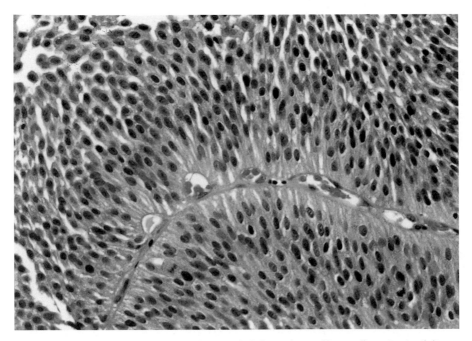

FIG. 3.15. Higher magnification of papillary urothelial neoplasm of low malignant potential seen in Figure 3.14.

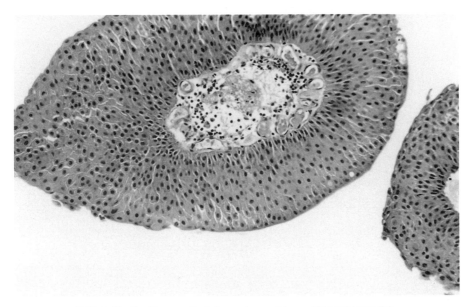

FIG. 3.16. Papillary urothelial neoplasm of low malignant potential.

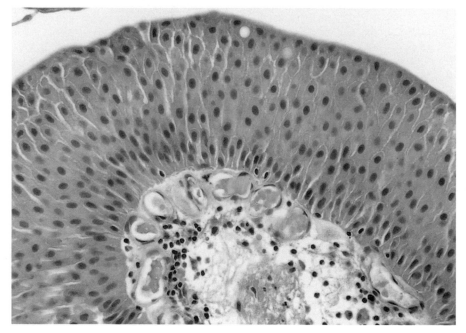

FIG. 3.17. Higher magnification of papillary urothelial neoplasm of low malignant potential seen in Figure 3.16.

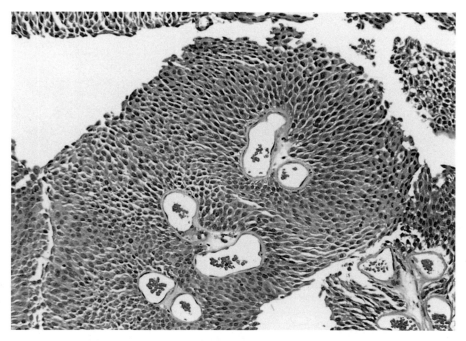

FIG. 3.18. Papillary urothelial neoplasm of low malignant potential.

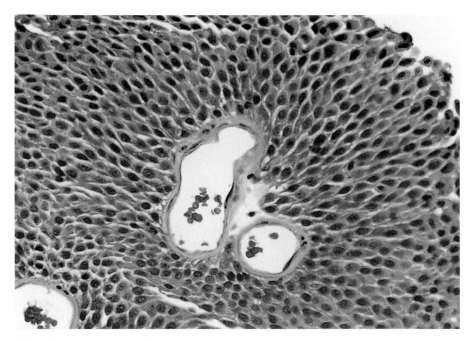

FIG. 3.19. Higher magnification of papillary urothelial neoplasm of low malignant potential seen in Figure 3.18.

lesion (e.g., papilloma) diagnosed, so the patient might be followed up more closely. The prognoses of these lesions and other papillary tumors in the WHO(2003)/ISUP system are discussed later.

PUNLMPs at low power differ from papillomas by having thicker urothelium. Otherwise, there are no architectural abnormalities, because the lesion has no loss of polarity (presence of order). Cytologically, PUNLMPs have a monotonous appearance, with each cell being virtually identical to each other. At most, nuclei are slightly enlarged and more crowded relative to those in normal urothelial nuclei. Nuclear grooves, a feature of normal urothelium, may be seen in these tumors and in papillomas, but not in higher grade lesions. Nucleoli are either absent or inconspicuous. The chromatin is uniformly even without the scattered hyperchromatic nuclei seen in low-grade papillary carcinoma. Mitoses are infrequent and usually limited to the basal layer. Occasional cases of PUNLMP have inverted features (efigs 277–283).

Low-Grade Papillary Carcinoma

To simplify the WHO (1973) system and avoid an intermediate cancer grade group (WHO 1973 grade 2), which is often the default diagnosis for many pathologists, the WHO(2003)/ISUP system classifies papillary urothelial carcinoma into only two grades. Additional reasons for having a two-tier grading system are described under "Papillary Urothelial Neoplasms: Prognosis Across Different Grades." Low-grade papillary urothelial carcinoma exhibits an overall orderly appearance but has minimal variability in architecture and cytologic features, which are easily recognizable at scanning magnification (Figs. 3.20–3.25) (Color Plate 3) (efigs 284–332). When analyzing for the presence of order versus disorder, it is preferable to assess only those fibrovascular cores that have been cut perpendicular to the long axis of the papillary frond, because tangential sections near the base of the frond may be misleading. This applies to all papillary urothelial tumors, including PUNLMPs. It is common to see fusion of adjacent papillae, a feature that may lead to overgrading because of its appearance of disorder.

Variability in polarity, nuclear size, shape, and chromatin texture are minimal but comprise the hallmarks of the cytologic atypia seen in low-grade papillary urothelial carcinoma. Mitotic figures are infrequent. Although mitoses may be seen at any level of the urothelium, they are usually limited to the lower half. Among these features, the finding of scattered hyperchromatic nuclei and scattered "typical" mitotic figures best distinguishes this lesion from PUNLMP. Occasionally one sees similar cytologic features in thickened urothelium adjacent to a papillary neoplasm (efigs 329, 330).

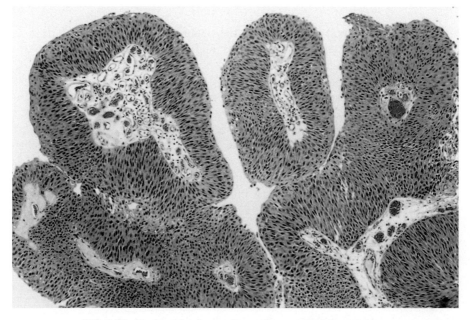

FIG. 3.20. Noninvasive low-grade papillary urothelial carcinoma.

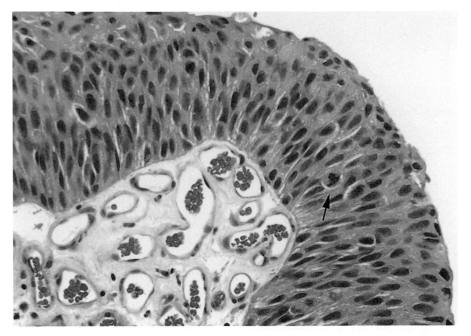

FIG. 3.21. Higher magnification of noninvasive low-grade papillary urothelial carcinoma seen in Figure 3.20. Note mitotic figure (*arrow*) midway up the urothelium.

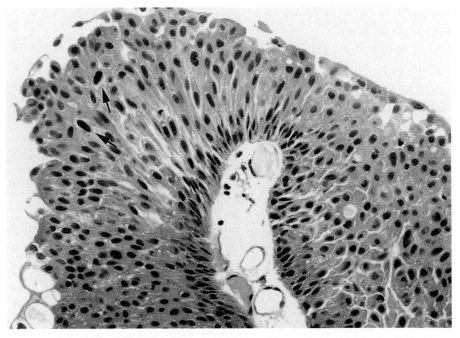

FIG. 3.22. Noninvasive low-grade papillary urothelial carcinoma. Note scattered hyperchromatic nuclei (*arrows*) and irregularity of size and shape of nuclei.

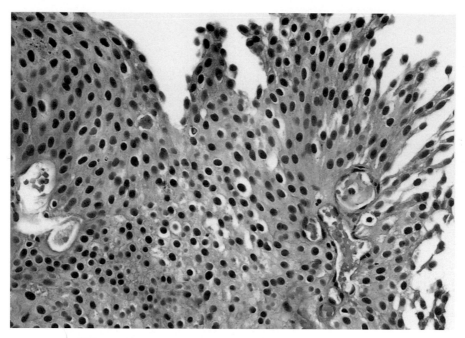

FIG. 3.23. Noninvasive low-grade papillary urothelial carcinoma.

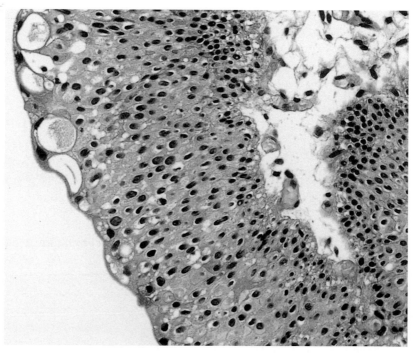

FIG. 3.24. Noninvasive low-grade papillary urothelial carcinoma.

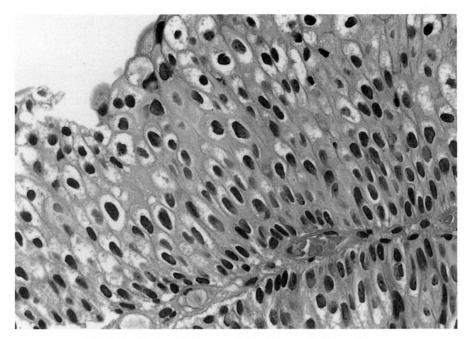

FIG. 3.25. Noninvasive low-grade papillary urothelial carcinoma.

High-Grade Papillary Carcinoma

High-grade papillary urothelial carcinomas are characterized by a disorderly appearance resulting from marked architectural and cytologic abnormalities, for the most part recognizable at low magnification (Figs. 3.26–3.34) (efigs 333–398). Architecturally, the cells are irregularly oriented and disorganized. Cellular pleomorphism ranges from moderate to marked. The nuclear chromatin tends to be clumped and nucleoli may be prominent and irregular. Mitotic figures, including atypical forms, may be frequently seen at all levels of the urothelium. A single papillary urothelial neoplasm may contain a spectrum of cytologic and architectural abnormalities. In tumors with variable histology, the tumor should be graded according to the highest grade, although current practice is to ignore minuscule areas of higher grade tumor. Studies are needed to determine how significant a minor component must be in order to have an impact on prognosis.

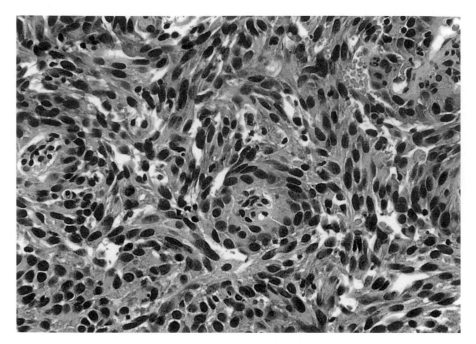

FIG. 3.26. Noninvasive high-grade papillary urothelial carcinoma.

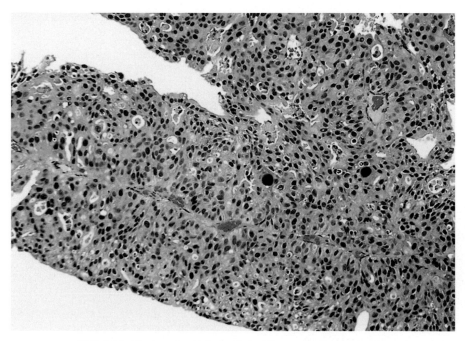

FIG. 3.27. Noninvasive high-grade papillary urothelial carcinoma.

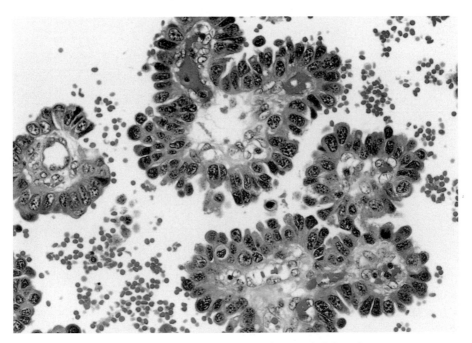

FIG. 3.28. Noninvasive high-grade papillary urothelial carcinoma.

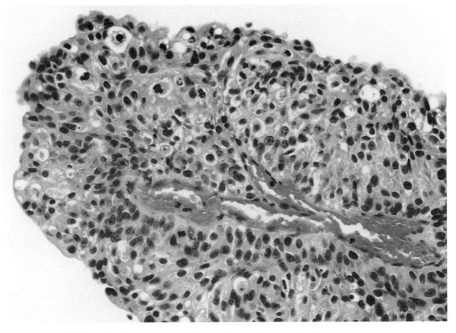

FIG. 3.29. Noninvasive high-grade papillary urothelial carcinoma.

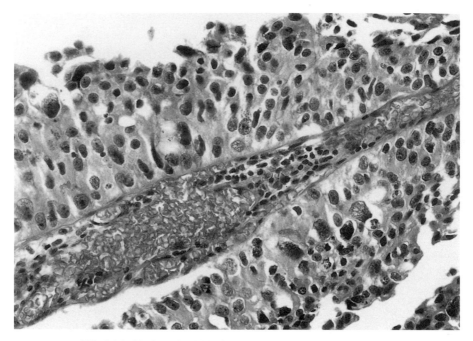

FIG. 3.30. Noninvasive high-grade papillary urothelial carcinoma.

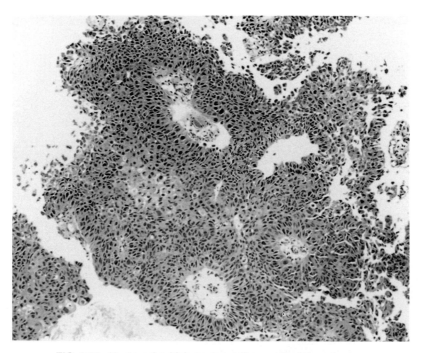

FIG. 3.31. Noninvasive high-grade papillary urothelial carcinoma.

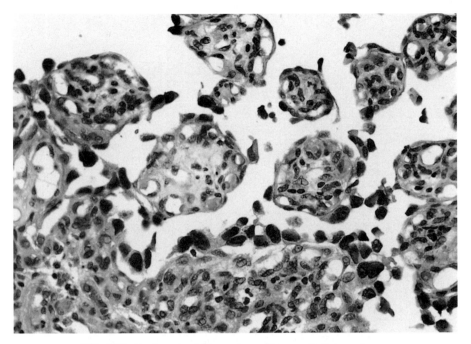

FIG. 3.32. Noninvasive high-grade papillary urothelial carcinoma.

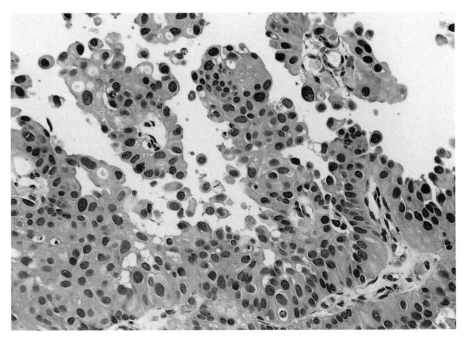

FIG. 3.33. Noninvasive high-grade papillary urothelial carcinoma.

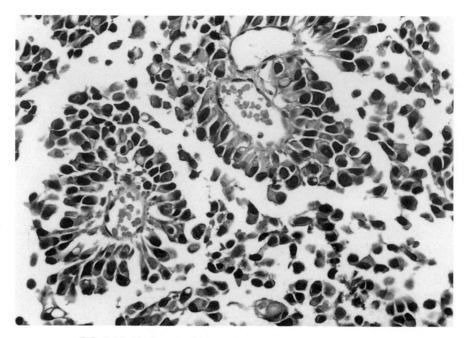

FIG. 3.34. Noninvasive high-grade papillary urothelial carcinoma.

Papillary Urothelial Neoplasms: Early Controversy

One of the earliest articles in which the WHO(2003)/ISUP system was applied led to controversy regarding the classification system (15). This article was submitted before the WHO(2003)/ISUP classification system was published and before there were detailed illustrations or descriptions on how to classify tumors using the new system. In the article, lesions that were formerly called WHO (1973) grade 1 were designated as PUNLMP. As described earlier, if these lesions were analyzed using the WHO(2003)/ISUP classification system, a subset of these tumors may not have been classified as PUNLMP, but would be diagnosed as low-grade urothelial carcinomas. According to the article, tumors classified as PUNLMP had a significant risk of recurrence, progression, and death from bladder cancer. This article has been cited as an argument against the use of the WHO(2003)/ISUP system.

Papillary Urothelial Neoplasms: Prognosis Across Different Grades

In 2000, Desai and colleagues used the WHO(2003)/ISUP system to correlate lesions with prognosis (16). Although papillomas did not progress or recur, and LMP tumors recurred but did not progress, low-grade and, to a greater extent,

TABLE 3.3. *Relation of World Health Organization/International Society of Urological Pathology grades to progression*

	Papilloma (n = 8)	PUNLMP (n = 8)	Low grade (n = 42)	High grade (n = 62)
Recurrence	0%	33.3%	64.1%	56.4%
Any stage progression	0%	0%	10.5%	27.1%
Lamina propria invasion	0%	0%	2.6%	8.3%
Detrusor muscle invasion	0%	0%	5.3%	6.3%
Metastases/death	0%	0%	10.6%	25.0%

PUNLMP, papillary urothelial neoplasms of low malignant potential.
From Desai S, Lim SD, Jiminez RE, et al. Relationship of cytokeratin 20 and CD44 protein expression with WHO/ISUP grade in pTa and pT1 papillary urothelial neoplasia. *Mod Pathol* 2000;13:1315–1323, with permission.

high-grade carcinomas experienced progression and, in some cases, patients died (Table 3.3).

The largest study to date using the WHO(2003)/ISUP classification system is that by Holmang and colleagues (17) (Table 3.4). Patients with PUNLMP tumors at last follow-up mostly had no evidence of disease with a small percentage of patients having tumor at last follow-up, yet no one died of disease. In contrast, patients with low-grade carcinoma had an increased risk of tumor being present at last follow-up, in addition to a small percentage of patients dying of disease. Patients with high-grade carcinoma had a larger (16%) risk of dying of disease.

In analyzing tumors using the WHO(2003)/ISUP classification system for p53 expression and proliferation as measured by KI67, an increase in P53 expression from 0.4% to 2.9% to 25.7% was documented in cases of LMP, low-grade carcinoma, and high-grade carcinoma, respectively (18). Proliferation also increased among the three grades from 2.5% to 7.3%, to 15.7%. The progression rates for WHO(2003)/ISUP papilloma, PUNLMP, low-grade, and high grade carcinomas were 0%, 8%, 13%, and 51%, respectively, in another study (19).

TABLE 3.4. *Relation of World Health Organization/International Society of Urological Pathology grades to progression*

	PUNLMP (n = 95)	Low grade (n = 160)	High grade (n = 108)
No evidence of disease	94%	76%	67%
Alive with disease	3%	10%	9%
Dead with disease	1%	6%	7%
Dead of disease	0%	4%	16%
No follow-up	2%	4%	1%

PUNLMP, papillary urothelial neoplasms of low malignant potential.
From Holmang S, Andius P, Hedelin H, et al. Stage progression in TA papillary urothelial tumors: relationship to grade, immunohistochemical expression of tumor markers, mitotic frequency and DNA ploidy. *J Urol* 2001;165:1124–1130, with permission.

Papillary Urothelial Neoplasms of Low Malignant Potential Versus Low-Grade Carcinoma

In 2001, Alsheikh focused on the differences between PUNLMPs and low-grade carcinomas (20). Whereas only five of 20 (25%) of the PUNLMPs recurred, 14 of 29 (48.2%) of low-grade carcinomas recurred. Of the two patients whose lesions progressed to high-grade muscle invasive carcinoma, both were initially low-grade carcinomas. Also, one patient's lesion progressed to CIS who also initially had low-grade carcinoma. Pich and coworkers also focused their investigations on differences between PUNLMPs and low-grade carcinomas (21). Differences in recurrence were noted between PUNLMPs and low-grade cancers with recurrence rates of 47.4% and 76.7%, respectively. Whereas none of the PUNLMPs progressed, 11.6% of the low-grade carcinomas progressed. The recurrence-free interval between PUNLMPs and low-grade carcinomas was also different, with 76- and 15-month recurrence-free intervals, respectively. Differences were also noted between the two WHO(2003)/ISUP grades in their p53 expression, mitoses, and MIB1 positivity. In a conflicting study, Oosterhuis and colleagues found no statistically significant differences in progression between LMP and low-grade carcinoma (22).

Despite most studies demonstrating prognostic differences between PUNLMP and low-grade carcinoma when evaluated by experts, Murphy and coworkers found that practitioners could not reliably distinguish between PUNLMPs and low-grade carcinomas, yet could discriminate between PUNLMP/low-grade carcinoma versus high-grade carcinoma (23). It is anticipated that with further use of the system the reproducibility will improve. Even if practitioners have difficulty with this differential diagnosis, it is still useful in that it provides a noncancerous diagnosis for a group of patients with indolent disease who would otherwise be classified as having cancer. This is especially useful for the younger patient with a newly diagnosed noninvasive papillary tumor that would not fulfill the criteria of papilloma because of its thicker urothelium.

Carcinomas: Two Grades or Three?

Another controversial area in the WHO(2003)/ISUP classification system is that carcinomas are dichotomized as low or high grade, whereas in the WHO (1999) system, high-grade carcinomas are divided into two grades (grade 2 and grade 3). Valid arguments supporting the subdivision of high-grade cancer into two grades are as follows:

1. High-grade cancer has a spectrum of atypia with some cases showing marked anaplasia.
2. Cases with marked anaplasia have a worse prognosis than other high-grade cancers.

One argument against subdividing high-grade cancers is that high-grade non-invasive papillary cancers with marked anaplasia comprise only a small percentage of noninvasive papillary cancers. In Holmang's study, of the 363 noninvasive papillary carcinomas, only 13 (3.6%) were classified as WHO (1973) grade 3, compared with 28% of the cases classified as high-grade carcinoma by the WHO(2003)/ISUP system (17). These data are similar to ours in which only 4.5% of noninvasive papillary tumors were WHO (1973) grade 3 compared with 21.6% classified as WHO(2003)/ISUP high grade (19). There are so few WHO (1973) grade 3 noninvasive papillary carcinomas because most cases of WHO (1973) grade 3 are aggressive tumors in which there is already coexisting invasive cancer. Because patients with high-grade noninvasive papillary carcinoma are not treated with definitive therapy (e.g., cystectomy), the goal should not be to restrict the high-risk group to a small population but to expand it to be more inclusive of all patients at significant risk of progression so that they can be monitored closely.

The other problem with dividing high-grade cancers into grades 2 and 3 is that there is considerable confusion for pathologists to recognize that grades 2 and 3 cancer from the WHO (1973) system are not the same as grades 2 and 3 cancer in the WHO (1999) system. Because pathologists are familiar with using grade 2 from the older WHO (1973) system to denote intermediate grade cancer, grade 2 tumors in the WHO (1999) system will include many tumors that would be classified as low-grade cancer by the current WHO(2003)/ISUP grading system.

CONCLUSIONS

The potential accomplishments of the WHO(2003)/ISUP system are as follows:

1. Establishment of uniform terminology and common definitions for urologic pathologists.
2. Establishment of detailed criteria of various preneoplastic conditions and various grades of tumor, leading to greater interobserver reproducibility.
3. Correlation with urine cytology terminology, facilitating cytohistologic correlation and making it easier for urologists to manage patients.
4. Creation of a category of tumor that identifies a tumor with a negligible risk of progression (PUNLMP), whereby patients avoid the label of having cancer, which has psychosocial and financial implications. Neither is benign lesion diagnosed in these patients, so they may still be followed up closely.
5. Identification of a distinct group of patients (high-grade papillary urothelial carcinoma and CIS) who would be ideal candidates for intravesical therapy.
6. Identification of a larger group of patients at high risk for progression for urologists to follow up more closely.
7. Removal of ambiguity in diagnostic categories in WHO 1973 system (e.g., TCC grade I-II, TCC grade II-III).
8. Stratification of bladder tumors into prognostically significant categories.

REFERENCES

1. Epstein JI, Amin MB, Reuter VE, et al. The World Health Organization/International Society of Urological Pathology consensus classification of urothelial (transitional cell) neoplasms of the urinary bladder. *Am J Surg Pathol* 1998;12:1435–1448.
2. Taylor DC, Bhagavan BS, Larsen MP, et al. Papillary urothelial hyperplasia. A precursor to papillary neoplasms. *Am J Surg Pathol* 1996;20:1481–1488.
3. Swierczinski SL, Epstein JI. Prognostic significance of atypical papillary urothelial hyperplasia. *Hum Pathol* 2002;33;512–517.
4. Eble JN, Young RH. Benign and low-grade papillary lesions of the urinary bladder: a review of the papilloma-papillary carcinoma controversy and a report of 5 typical papillomas. *Semin Diagn Pathol* 1989;6:351–371.
5. Broders AC. Epithelium of the genito-urinary organs. *Ann Surg* 1922;75:574–604.
6. Bergkvist A, Ljungqvist A, Moberger G. Classification of bladder tumours based on the cellular pattern. *Acta Chir Scand* 1965;130:371–378.
7. Mostofi FK, Sobin LH, Torloni H. *Histological typing of urinary bladder tumours. International classification of tumors 19*. Geneva: World Health Organization, 1973.
8. Ooms ECM, Anderson WAAD, Alons CL, et al. Analysis of the performance of pathologists in the grading of bladder tumors. *Hum Pathol* 1983;14:140–143.
9. Jordan AM, Weingarten J, Murphy WM. Transitional cell neoplasms of the urinary bladder. Can biologic potential be predicted from histologic grading? *Cancer* 1987;60:2766–2774.
10. Malmström P-U, Busch C, Norlén BJ. Recurrence, progression and survival in bladder cancer: a retrospective analysis of 232 patients with 5-year follow-up. *Scand J Urol Nephrol* 1987;21:185–195.
11. Abel PD, Henderson D, Bennett, et al. Differing interpretations by pathologists of the pT category and grade of transitional cell cancer of the bladder. *Br J Urol* 1988;62:339–342.
12. Carbin B-E, Ekman P, Gustafson H, et al. Grading of human urothelial carcinoma based on nuclear atypia and mitotic frequency. II: Prognostic importance. *J Urol* 1991;145:972–976.
13. Pathology and genetics of tumours of the urinary system and male genital organs. In: Eble JN, Sauter G, Epstein JI, et al, eds. *World Health classification of tumours*. Lyon: IARC Press, 2003.
14. McKenney JK, Amin MB, Young RH. Urothelial (transitional cell) papilloma of the urinary bladder: a clinicopathologic study of 26 cases. *Mod Pathol* 2003;16:623–629.
15. Cheng L, Newman RM, Bostwick DG. Papillary urothelial neoplasms of low malignant potential. *Cancer* 1999;86:2102–2108.
16. Desai S, Lim SD, Jiminez RE, et al. Relationship of cytokeratin 20 and CD44 protein expression with WHO/ISUP grade in pTa and pT1 papillary urothelial neoplasia. *Mod Pathol* 2000;13:1315–1323.
17. Holmang S, Andius P, Hedelin H, et al. Stage progression in TA papillary urothelial tumors: relationship to grade, immunohistochemical expression of tumor markers, mitotic frequency and DNA ploidy. *J Urol* 2001;165:1124–1130.
18. Cina SJ, Lancaster-Weiss KJ, Lecksell K, et al. Correlation of KI-67 and p53 with the new World Health Organization/International Society of Urological Pathology classification system for urothelial neoplasia. *Arch Pathol Lab Med* 2001;125:646–651.
19. Samaratunga H, Makarov, DV, Epstein JI. Comparison of WHO/ISUP and WHO classification of non-invasive papillary urothelial neoplasms for risk of progression. *Urology* 2002;60:315–319.
20. Alsheikh A, Mohamedali Z, Jones E, et al. Comparison of the WHO/ISUP classification and cytokeratin 20 expression in predicting the behavior of low-grade papillary urothelial tumors. *Mod Pathol* 2001;14:267–272.
21. Pich A, Chiusa L, Formiconi A, et al. Biologic differences between noninvasive papillary urothelial neoplasms of low malignant potential and low grade (grade 1) papillary carcinomas of the bladder. *Am J Surg Pathol* 2001;25:1528–1533.
22. Oosterhuis JEA, Schapers RFM, Janssen-Heijnen MLG, et al. Histological grading of papillary urothelial carcinoma of the bladder: prognostic value of the 1998 WHO/ISUP classification system and comparison with conventional grading systems. *J Clin Pathol* 2002;55:900–905.
23. Murphy WM, Takezawa K, Maruniak NA. Interobserver discrepancy using the 1998 World Health Organization/International Society of Urologic Pathology classification of urothelial neoplasms. Practical choices for patient care. *J Urol* 2002;68:968–972.

4

Urothelial Neoplasms with Inverted Growth Patterns

UROTHELIAL NEOPLASMS (EXCLUDING INVERTED PAPILLOMAS)

Urothelial neoplasms exhibit two patterns of endophytic or inverted growth: (a) broad front verrucous carcinoma-like growth and (b) inverted papilloma-like growth (1). The two patterns may coexist, and either pattern may or may not be associated with frank stromal invasion. In broad-front growth, like verrucous carcinoma, broad bulbous tongues of neoplastic urothelium extend deep into the lamina propria and sometimes may reach up to the muscularis propria. In our opinion, despite the deep penetration, invasion is not present if the basement membrane is smooth, and the likelihood of metastasis is minimal. If, however, there is irregularity of the basement membrane of the bulbous endophytic tongues of broad-front growth, and if there is retraction artifact, desmoplasia, or other features suggestive of destructive invasion, the tumor must be designated as invasive (1).

In tumors with inverted papilloma-like growth, the basic configuration is like inverted papilloma, that is, endophytic, expansile growth with or without peripheral palisading of basaloid cells. In contrast to inverted papilloma, inverted urothelial carcinomas have a variable proportion of exophytic component, and the ramifying cords and trabeculae are less uniform and sometimes solid without polarity (Figs. 4.1–4.6) (efigs 399–414) (Table 4.1). If the endophytic component has markedly thickened but otherwise cytologically unremarkable cords and the exophytic component is similar, the designation of inverted urothelial neoplasm of low malignant potential is appropriate. If there is cytologic atypia, depending on the grade, the tumors would be designated as inverted (i.e., not with invasion) urothelial carcinoma, low grade or high grade. As in broad-front verrucous carcinoma-like growth, inverted papilloma-like destructive invasion may be present in tumors with endophytic growth. In such a case, diagnostic terminology such as *urothelial carcinoma with endophytic growth, high grade, with invasion into lamina propria* may be used.

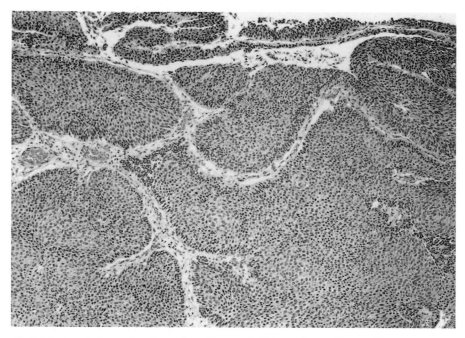

FIG. 4.1. Inverted growth pattern of papillary urothelial neoplasm of low malignant potential.

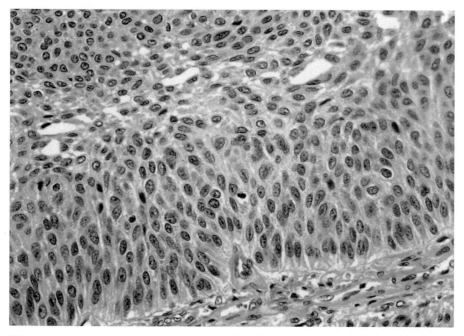

FIG. 4.2. Inverted growth pattern of papillary urothelial neoplasm of low malignant potential with thicker columns of urothelium than inverted papilloma (higher magnification of Figure 4.1).

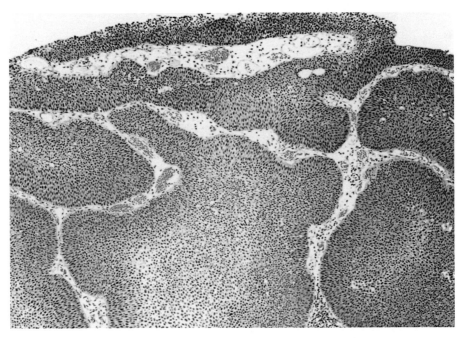

FIG. 4.3. Noninvasive low-grade papillary urothelial carcinoma with inverted growth pattern.

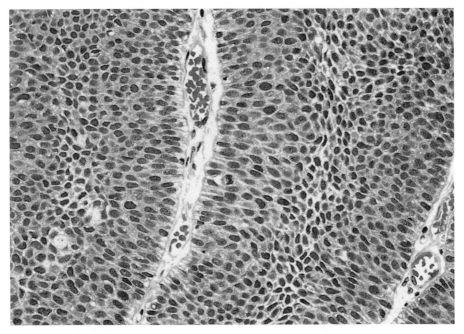

FIG. 4.4. Noninvasive low-grade papillary urothelial carcinoma with inverted growth pattern (higher magnification of Figure 4.3).

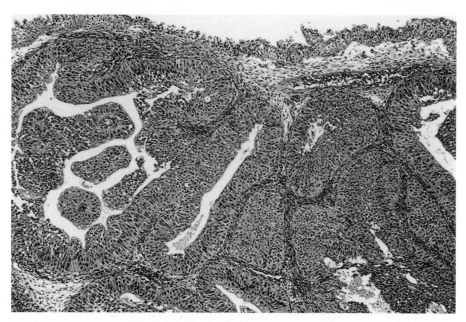

FIG. 4.5. Noninvasive low-grade papillary urothelial carcinoma with inverted growth pattern. Note true papillary frond formation and mitotic figure.

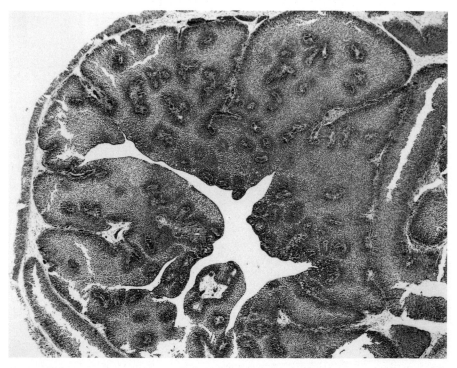

FIG. 4.6. Noninvasive low-grade papillary urothelial carcinoma with inverted growth pattern. Note true papillary frond formation.

TABLE 4.1. *Differences between inverted papilloma and urothelial carcinoma with inverted papilloma-like growth*

	Inverted papilloma	Urothelial carcinoma with inverted papilloma-like growth
Surface	Smooth dome-shaped or focally exophytic, cytologically unremarkable, usually intact surface	Variable, usually exophytic papillary lesion
Growth pattern	Endophytic, expansile, sharply delineated lesion	Endophytic; may coexist with "verrucous carcinoma-like" inverted growth pattern; lesional circumscription variable
	Ramifying cords and trabeculae of even width	Ramifying cords and trabeculae with irregularity of width and with transition into solid areas
	Destructive invasion of lamina propria or muscularis propria absent by definition	Possible invasion into lamina propria or muscle
Cytologic features	Orderly polarized cells with tendency to spindle and palisade at the periphery	Maturation, spindling, or palisading minimal to absent
	Diffuse, severe cytologic atypia absent	Cytologic features are grade dependent (urothelial carcinoma, low grade or high grade)
Biologic potential	Benign, recurrences none	Recur (usually new occurrences) or progress (depends on grade and stage)

INVERTED UROTHELIAL PAPILLOMA

This is a benign tumor of the urinary bladder comprising less than 1% of urothelial neoplasms. Cystoscopically, they appear as solitary, raised, pedunculated, or, rarely, polypoid lesions with a smooth surface (2). Lesions occur in a wide age range of patients (10 to 94 years), with a peak frequency in the sixth and seventh decades; there is a striking male predilection (3,4). Tumor size varies from small (less than 3 cm) to large (up to 8 cm). Most lesions are solitary and present with hematuria.

Histologically, two variations have been described: trabecular and glandular (2). The trabecular type is the classic lesion that most pathologists think of when considering inverted papilloma, histologically showing cords and trabeculae of cells arising from a smooth surface and invaginating into the lamina propria (Figs. 4.7–4.14) (Color Plate 4) (efigs 415–456). Because these endophytic proliferations represent inversion of papillae, the periphery is composed of darker cells that are often palisaded (the basal cells), and the central portions show maturing cells occasionally with superficial cells lining central luminal spaces. The surrounding stroma is fibrotic and nonreactive without inflammation. Cytologic atypia is minimal to absent, although occasionally atypia of the degenerate type (smudged, hyperchromatic, occasionally multinucleated cells) may be pre-

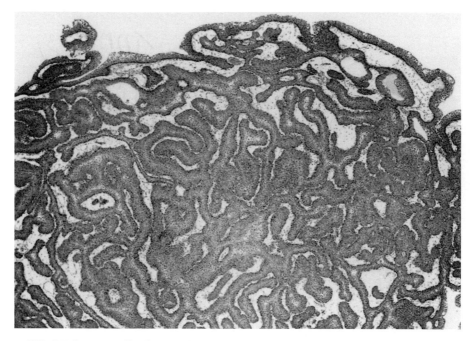

FIG. 4.7. Low magnification showing overall architecture of inverted urothelial papilloma.

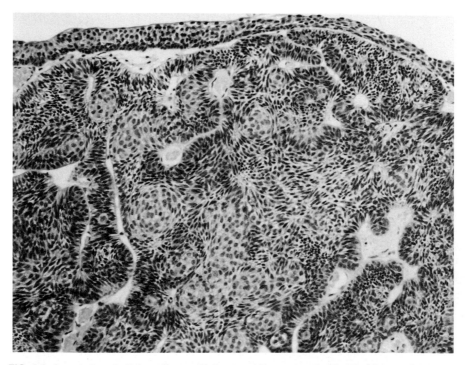

FIG. 4.8. Inverted urothelial papilloma with "squamoid" appearance of underlying anastomosing nests of urothelium.

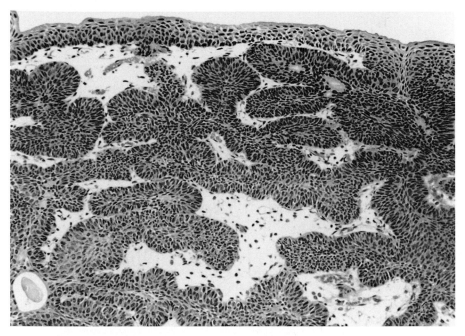

FIG. 4.9. Inverted urothelial papilloma with loose stroma lacking inflammation.

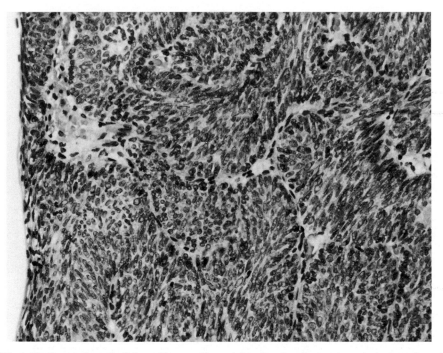

FIG. 4.10. Inverted urothelial papilloma with peripheral palisading and central streaming of urothelium in trabeculae.

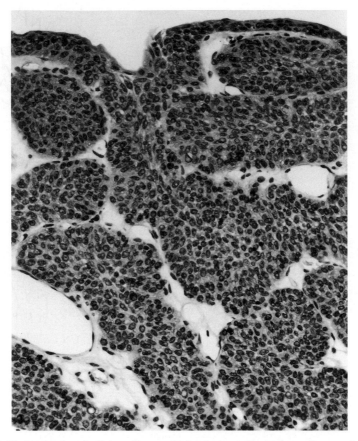

FIG. 4.11. Inverted urothelial papilloma with focal connection to the surface urothelium.

sent, albeit focally (Fig. 4.15) (efigs 457–459). Mitotic figures are rare and are only seen at the periphery of the trabeculae. The trabeculae are orderly, of relatively uniform width, with considerable ramifications and interanastomosis. Occasionally there may be marked von Brunn nest proliferation in the adjacent mucosa. Squamous metaplasia without keratinization may be seen. Paneth cell–like neuroendocrine differentiation is exceptionally rare (5). In our opinion, cases of the glandular subtype overlap in their morphology with florid cystitis cystica et glandularis and we do not use the term *inverted papilloma, glandular type*.

As in exophytic papillary neoplasms, inverted neoplasms may show a spectrum of differentiation within the same tumor such that a neoplasm may be composed of classic inverted papilloma histology with focal areas of inverted low malignant potential tumor histology, low-grade carcinoma, or even high-grade

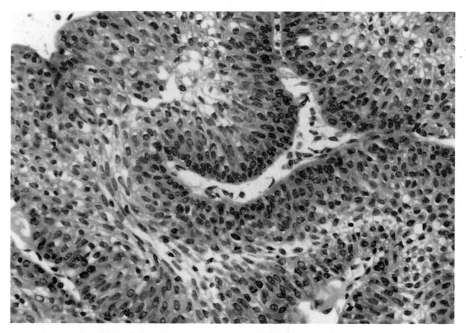

FIG. 4.12. Inverted urothelial papilloma with peripheral palisading and central streaming of urothelium in trabeculae.

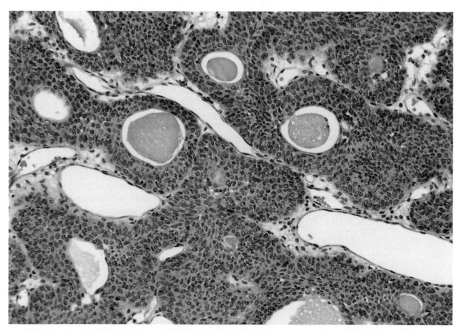

FIG. 4.13. Inverted urothelial papilloma with colloid cyst formation.

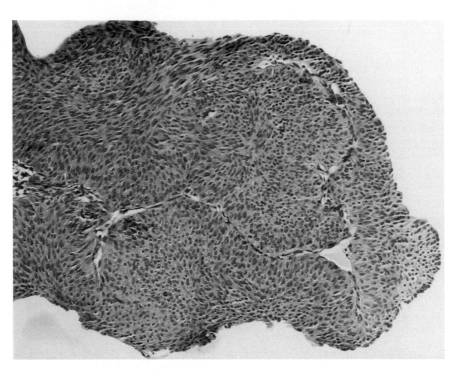

FIG. 4.14. Focal exophytic area in an otherwise classic inverted urothelial papilloma. Even though the area is exophytic, it lacks a true fibrovascular core and has an inverted growth pattern within the center of the polypoid focus.

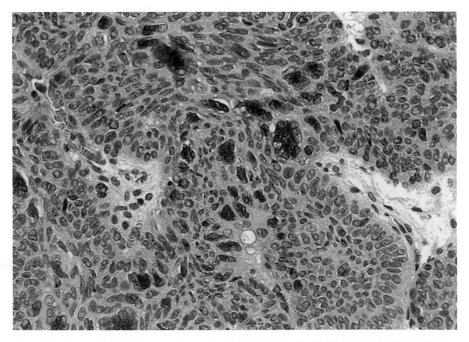

FIG. 4.15. Inverted urothelial papilloma with scattered atypical cells consisting of multinucleated and degenerative appearing nuclei.

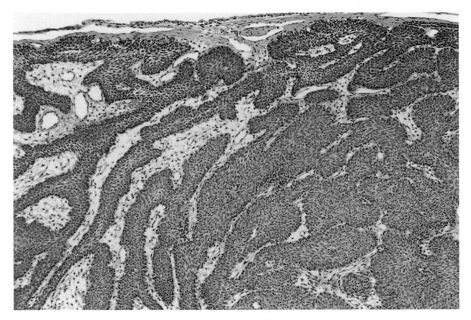

FIG. 4.16. Classic inverted urothelial papilloma.

carcinoma (Figs. 4.16, 4.17) (efigs 460–473). One of the authors (J.I.E.) has studied inverted papillomas with very focal atypia subdivided into the following groups: (a) areas containing prominent nucleoli, (b) foci with atypical squamous features, and (c) foci with areas of dysplasia, approaching the level of carcinoma in situ (efigs 474–481). To date, there has been no association with urothelial carcinomas in these individuals diagnosed with inverted papilloma and very focal atypia. The designation of these cases is controversial, whether they should be considered as inverted papillomas with focal atypia or as urothelial carcinomas arising in an inverted papilloma.

Three features are key to the recognition of inverted papilloma: (a) a relatively smooth surface with minimal to absent exophytic component, (b) lesional circumscription with a smooth base without obvious infiltration, and (c) minimal to absent cytologic atypia (5). In our opinion, a prominent exophytic component, considerable cytologic atypia (equivalent to low-grade or high-grade papillary urothelial carcinoma), irregularity of proliferating nests with solid areas, and obvious invasion would disqualify a lesion as being diagnosed as inverted papilloma. If the diagnosis of inverted papilloma is strictly defined in accordance with the criteria outlined, this lesion is benign with infrequent recurrences and progression. In our opinion, most cases reported as inverted papilloma with concurrent urothelial carcinoma represent the inverted pattern of urothelial carcinoma.

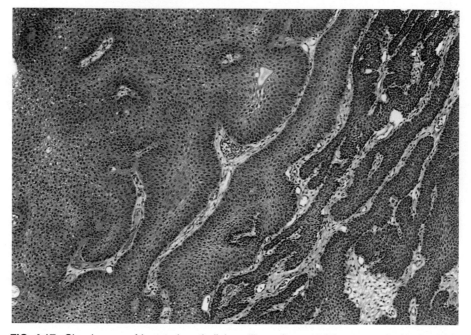

FIG. 4.17. Classic area of inverted urothelial papilloma (lower right) compared with the thickened urothelium more consistent with an inverted growth pattern of papillary urothelial neoplasm of low malignant potential (upper left) (same case as shown in Figure 4.16).

REFERENCES

1. Amin MB, Gomez JA, Young RH. Urothelial transitional cell carcinoma with endophytic growth patterns: a discussion of patterns of invasion and problems associated with assessment of invasion in 18 cases. *Am J Surg Pathol* 1997;21:1057–1068.
2. Kunze E, Schauer A, Schmitt M. Histology and histogenesis of two different types of inverted urothelial papillomas. *Cancer* 1983;51:348–358.
3. Yagi H, Igawa M, Shiina H, et al. Inverted papilloma of the urinary bladder in a girl. *Urol Int* 1999; 63:258–260.
4. DeMeester LJ, Farrow GM, Utz DC. Inverted papilloma of the urinary bladder. *Cancer* 1975;36: 505–513.
5. Summers DE, Rushin JM, Frazier HA, et al. Inverted papilloma of the urinary bladder with granular eosinophilic cells. An unusual neuroendocrine variant. *Arch Pathol Lab Med* 1991;115:802–806.

5

Invasive Urothelial Carcinoma

Invasion in urothelial carcinoma may arise at the base of a papillary neoplasm or within it. It can also be seen as microinvasive or invasive disease in association with carcinoma in situ, or CIS (CIS with invasion). In some cases, a precursor lesion is not seen, presumably because it has been destroyed by surface ulceration associated with the invasive carcinoma.

USUAL OR CONVENTIONAL TYPE OF UROTHELIAL CARCINOMA

Invasive urothelial carcinoma may present as a polypoid, sessile, ulcerated or infiltrative lesion in which the neoplastic cells invade the bladder wall as nests, cords, trabeculae, small clusters, or single cells that are often separated by a desmoplastic stroma. The tumor sometimes grows in a more diffuse, sheetlike pattern, but even in these cases, focal nests and clusters are generally present. Occasionally, carcinomas are associated with a pronounced chronic inflammatory cell infiltrate, which partially or substantially obscures the underlying tumor cells. The neoplastic cells in these typical or conventional patterns of invasive urothelial carcinoma are usually of moderate size and have modest amounts of pale to eosinophilic cytoplasm (Figs. 5.1–5.3). Sometimes tumors with a more nestlike architecture, eosinophilic cytoplasm in tumor cells, and prominent stromal vascularity between nests may mimic a paraganglioma (see Chapter 12). In some tumors, the cytoplasm is more abundant and may be clear or strikingly eosinophilic. The presence of clear cells, with rare exceptions, is focal, and should not lead to the diagnosis of clear cell adenocarcinoma, which has a very typical histology. Invasive tumors are invariably high grade, although there is a spectrum of some cases exhibiting marked anaplasia; focal tumor giant cell formation may be seen. Only a small minority of invasive urothelial carcinomas have a low-grade histology (see Chapter 6 for a description of nested variant of urothelial carcinoma); however, the outcome is not determined by tumor grade but rather by stage. By the World Health Organization 2003/International Society of Urological Pathologists [WHO(2003)/ISUP] classification, invasive tumors are graded as low grade and high grade. Features indicative of the urothe-

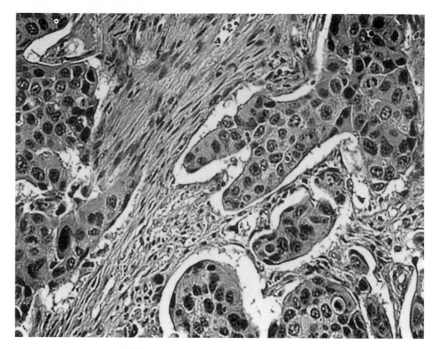

FIG. 5.1. Invasive urothelial carcinoma.

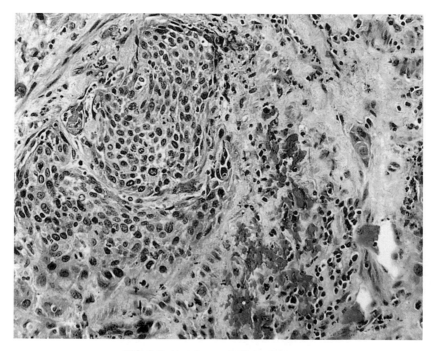

FIG. 5.2. Invasive urothelial carcinoma.

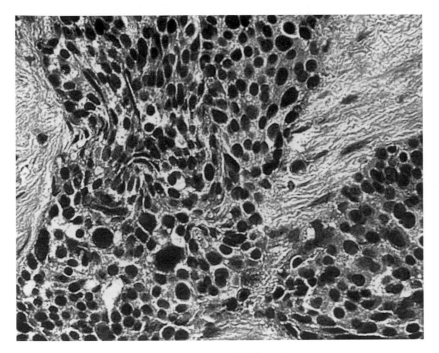

FIG. 5.3. Invasive urothelial carcinoma.

lial (transitional cell) character of cells of urothelial carcinoma include the presence of longitudinal nuclear grooves that are often appreciable in low-grade tumors, but are more focally present in high-grade tumors. Approximately 10% of urothelial carcinomas contain foci of glandular or squamous differentiation (see Chapters 8 and 9). Glandular differentiation is usually in the form of small tubular or glandlike spaces in conventional urothelial carcinoma (urothelial carcinoma with glandlike lumina) or as a histology similar to enteric adenocarcinoma. Rarely, a coexistent signet ring cell or mucinous component may be present. To designate squamous differentiation, one must see clear-cut evidence of squamous production (intracellular keratin, intercellular bridges, or keratin pearls), and the degree of squamous differentiation, when present, usually parallels the grade of the urothelial carcinoma. In general, urothelial carcinomas have a relatively nondescript appearance, which when viewed in isolation cannot be differentiated from poorly differentiated carcinomas of other types. Therefore, the presence of squamous or glandular differentiation in a poorly differentiated neoplasm suggests the possibility of urothelial differentiation. To designate a bladder tumor as pure squamous cell or pure adenocarcinoma, a pure histology of squamous cell carcinoma or adenocarcinoma is required. The presence of squamous and glandular differentiation in urothelial carcinomas has generally been thought of as lacking any clinical significance. In stage-matched cases, the outcome of typical urothelial carcinoma is similar to those with aberrant differentiation (1). However, some studies have suggested that these variants may be more resistant to chemotherapy or radiation therapy than pure urothelial carcinoma, but this has not been confirmed (2,3). From a practical viewpoint, we do make note of prominent squamous or glandular differentiation in urothelial carcinoma by using diagnostic terminology such as "invasive urothelial carcinoma," "invading muscularis propria," and "with prominent squamous (40%) and glandular (25%) differentiation." In cases of metastatic tumor, knowledge of the presence and percentage of divergent differentiation may be useful to facilitate comparison with the primary.

A subset of invasive urothelial carcinomas may exhibit vascular invasion. This parameter should be diagnosed with care, because invasive urothelial carcinomas, particularly those with limited or early invasion, frequently show retraction artifact, which mimics vascular–lymphatic invasion. In two studies, only 14% and 40% of cases originally diagnosed with vascular invasion on the basis of morphology could be proven by immunohistochemistry (4,5). Criteria for recognition of vascular invasion are outlined later in this chapter.

In addition to the morphology described earlier, invasive urothelial carcinoma has a propensity for myriad other patterns of divergent differentiation (e.g., small cell carcinoma, sarcomatoid carcinoma) or variation in histology (micropapillary, microcystic, nested) in approximately 10% of cases. These are described in detail in Chapter 6.

STAGING OF BLADDER CANCER

Stage is the most powerful prognostic indicator in urothelial carcinoma and is a major defining parameter in the management of this disease (1). The TNM (tumor, node, metastasis) staging system defines T1 tumors as those invading into the lamina propria but not the muscularis propria (6). Even though several studies have shown that T1 tumors bear a less favorable prognosis than Ta (noninvasive) neoplasms (7–9), clinically Ta and T1 tumors are usually lumped together by urologists under the term *superficial* bladder tumors, partially because these two stages traditionally have been managed conservatively. Another possible factor contributing to the clinician's rationale in grouping Ta and T1 tumors as superficial is the pathologists' inability to always accurately recognize lamina propria invasion (10,11). Contemporary series in which great care was taken to classify Ta and T1 correctly have shown clear differences in progression rates (12,13). On the contrary, tumors with involvement of the muscularis propria and beyond (pT2-4, or *invasive* tumors) are usually managed with aggressive surgical therapy (i.e., cystectomy) or radiation therapy with or without adjuvant therapy.

Before discussing lamina propria (T1) and muscularis propria (T2 and T2+) invasion, it is important to be aware of the type of specimens encountered in bladder pathology and some histologic aspects of the bladder wall that are pertinent for the discussion of invasion.

Most small bladder tumors (usually less than 1 cm in size) can frequently be excised by cold cup biopsies. This procedure yields specimens in which the cellular architecture is mostly preserved and orientation is easier to maintain after embedding. The resulting hematoxylin and eosin sections show the urothelial neoplasm, the lamina propria, and often superficial muscularis propria with orientation maintained, thus facilitating assessment of invasion (14). Larger tumors (usually greater than 1 cm) usually require hot loop resection (transurethral resection of bladder tumor, or TURBT), in which the urologist attempts to include a generous sample of the underlying muscle layer to enable adequate pathologic staging. The specimens rendered by this procedure are often fragmented, heavily cauterized, and difficult to orient. Sections from these specimens are complicated by thermal artifact, tangential sectioning, and disruption of the tumor and normal architecture. While examining both types of specimens, it is important to note the presence or absence of muscularis propria in the specimen to assess involvement of it by neoplasia and to provide feedback to the urologist regarding adequacy of resection.

The subepithelial connective tissue is a compact layer of fibrovascular connective tissue. In most instances, it is divided by a thin layer of smooth muscle fibers (muscularis mucosae) into a lamina propria proper, which is superficial, and a submucosal layer, located between the muscularis mucosae and muscularis propria. These anatomic landmarks may be entirely replaced by dense connective tissue at sites of prior biopsy. It was not until the 1980s that the muscularis mucosae layer of the urinary bladder was described (15–17), alerting pathologists and urologists of the importance of recognizing it and differentiating it from the underlying compact smooth muscle bundles of muscularis propria. Muscularis mucosae fibers are usually thin, often discontinuous, wispy and wavy fascicles of smooth muscle, which are frequently associated with large-caliber blood vessels, and surrounded by loose fibroconnective tissue. Most studies have identified some degree of this layer in 94% to 100% of cystectomy specimens (16,17) and in approximately 18% to 83% of specimens from biopsies or TURBT (12,18). Muscularis propria fascicles, on the other hand, are usually thick and compact, divided into distinct bundles surrounded by perimysium. Occasionally, muscularis mucosae bundles undergo hypertrophy especially after biopsy or at the base of the tumor, and in such situations the distinction between muscularis mucosae and muscularis propria, especially in biopsy or TURBT specimens, may be difficult. The deep (outer half) muscularis propria often rest on the perivesical fat. The boundary between them is not abrupt. Fat is often present in the bladder wall; the frequency and amount increase from the superficial lamina propria to the deep lamina propria, and to the muscularis propria (19).

Diagnosis of Lamina Propria Invasion

Recognition of lamina propria invasion by urothelial carcinoma is occasionally one of the most challenging diagnoses in surgical pathology (20) (Figs.

5.4–5.9) (efigs 482–528). Often faced with distorted, cauterized, and tangentially sectioned specimens, the pathologist should follow strict criteria to diagnose lamina propria invasion (Table 5.1). While evaluating tumors for invasion, it is important to focus on the features discussed in the following paragraphs.

Histologic Grade of Tumor

Lamina propria invasion should be carefully sought in all high-grade papillary carcinomas. Although invasion is not a common finding in low-grade tumors, it is much more common in high-grade lesions. In our experience, more than 90% of pT1 tumors are high grade. Thus, even though clear-cut histologic signs of invasion are required for the diagnosis of invasion into lamina propria, regardless of grade, the level of suspicion should be higher in those cases with a high histologic grade.

Characteristics of Invading Epithelium

The invasive front of the neoplasm may show one of several features: single cells or irregularly shaped nests of tumor within the stroma, architectural

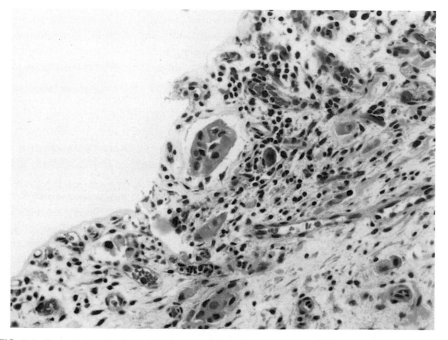

FIG. 5.4. Denuded urothelium with clusters of individual cells and small nests within lamina propria consistent with superficially infiltrating urothelial carcinoma.

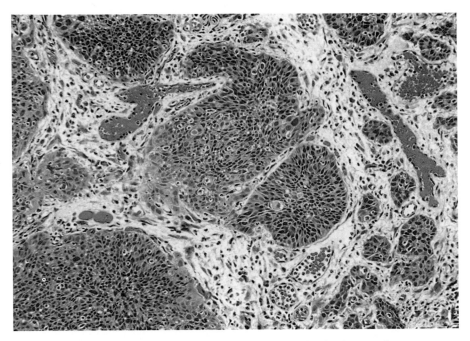

FIG. 5.5. Urothelial carcinoma superficially invading lamina propria.

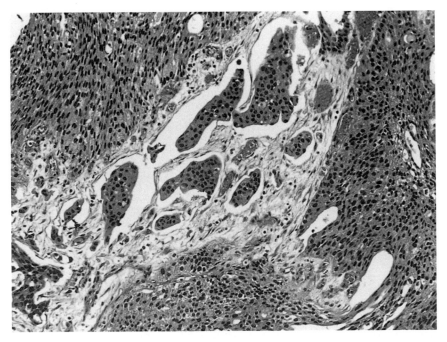

FIG. 5.6. Infiltrating urothelial carcinoma within lamina propria with prominent retraction artifact.

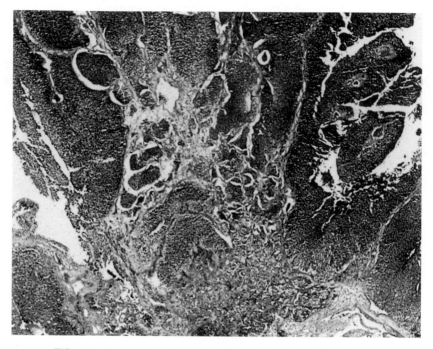

FIG. 5.7. Urothelial carcinoma invading base of papillary carcinoma.

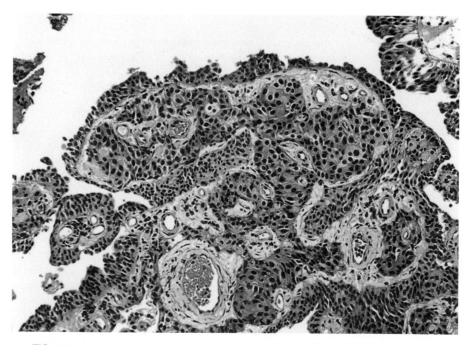

FIG. 5.8. Infiltrating urothelial carcinoma within stalk of papillary urothelial carcinoma.

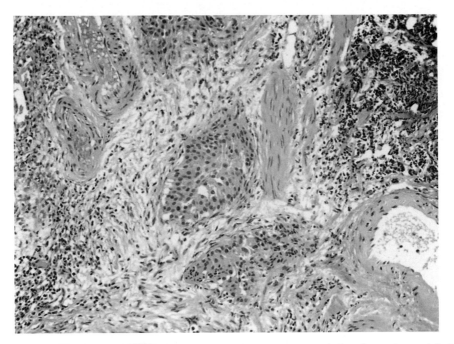

FIG. 5.9. Infiltrating urothelial carcinoma amongst thin, smooth muscle bundles and associated larger blood vessels typical of muscularis mucosae at the midlevel of the lamina propria.

TABLE 5.1. *Criteria for diagnosis of invasion into lamina propria by urothelial carcinoma*

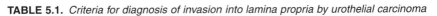

Histologic grade
    Invasion seen much more frequently, although not exclusively, in high-grade
        [WHO(2003)/ISUP classification] lesions.
Invading epithelium
    Irregularly shaped nests
    Single-cell infiltration
    Irregular or absent basement membrane
    Tentacular finger-like projections
    Invasive component with higher nuclear grade or more cytoplasm (or morphologically
        different) than overlying noninvasive component (paradoxical differentiation)
Stromal response
    Desmoplasia or sclerosis
    Retraction artifact
    Inflammation
    Myxoid stroma
    Pseudosarcomatous stroma
    Absent stromal response

WHO/ISUP, World Health Organization/International Society of Urological Pathology Consensus Classification of Bladder Tumors.

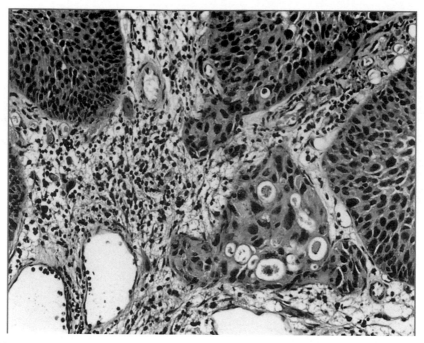

FIG. 5.10. Paradoxical differentiation with infiltrating nest of urothelial carcinoma in lamina propria showing abundant eosinophilic cytoplasm compared with overlying noninvasive high-grade papillary urothelial carcinoma.

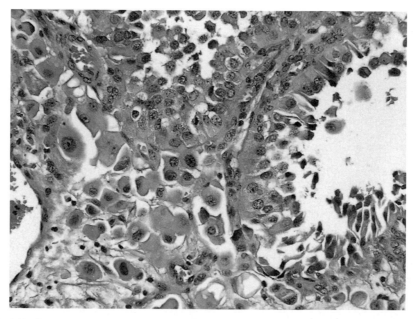

FIG. 5.11. Paradoxical differentiation with infiltrating single cells of urothelial carcinoma in lamina propria showing abundant eosinophilic cytoplasm compared with adjacent noninvasive high-grade papillary urothelial carcinoma.

complexity not conforming to the usual regularity of papillary neoplasms, or an irregular, disrupted, or absent basement membrane. Sometimes, tentacular or finger-like extensions can be seen arising from the base of the papillary tumor. Frequently, the invading nests appear morphologically different from the cells at the base of the noninvasive component of the tumor, with more abundant cytoplasm and often with a higher degree of pleomorphism (Figs. 5.10, 5.11). This phenomenon has been called *paradoxical differentiation* when seen at other sites such as the uterine cervix.

Stromal Response

The lamina propria may react to invasion in one or more of the following forms:

1. Desmoplastic or sclerotic stroma: The stroma may be cellular with spindled fibroblasts and variable collagenization, with or without inflammation.
2. Retraction artifact: In some cases, a retraction artifact that mimics vascular invasion is seen in tumors invading only superficially into the lamina propria (Fig. 5.12). Often this finding is focal and, in our opinion, is one of the early signs of invasion into lamina propria. It is especially conspicuous in

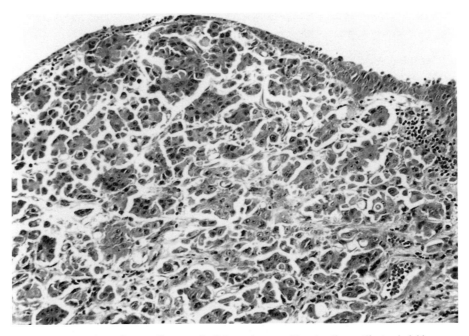

FIG. 5.12. Infiltrating micropapillary urothelial carcinoma with retraction artifact mimicking vascular invasion.

the micropapillary variant of urothelial carcinoma, but may be present in any invasive carcinoma.

3. Inflamed stroma: Invasion may elicit a brisk inflammatory response. The lamina propria is heavily infiltrated by numerous inflammatory cells that may obscure the interface between epithelium and stroma (Fig. 5.13). This makes recognition of small nests or single-cell invasion difficult to recognize.

4. Myxoid stroma: Loose and hypocellular stroma with a myxoid background may occasionally be seen in some cases of invasive urothelial carcinomas (Fig. 5.14).

5. Pseudosarcomatous stroma: Sometimes the tumor induces an exuberant spindle cell response, with proliferation of fibroblasts that may display significant, often alarming cellular atypia (21). This feature, although helpful in assessing for invasion, should not be mistaken for the spindle cell component of a biphasic sarcomatoid urothelial cancer (see Chapter 6). The proliferating stroma is usually nonexpansile, being limited to areas around the neoplasm, and is cytologically composed of cells that have a degenerate or smudged appearance on high-power examination.

6. Absent stromal response: Frequently the stromal response to invading carcinoma may be absent. This is particularly the case in areas of microinvasion.

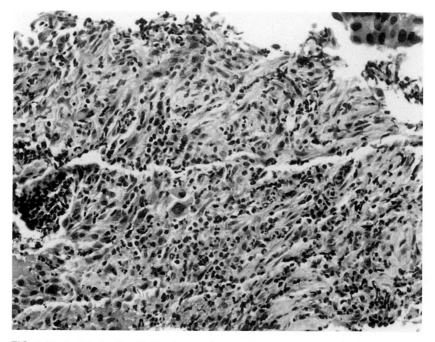

FIG. 5.13. Isolated cells of infiltrating carcinoma with associated intense inflammation.

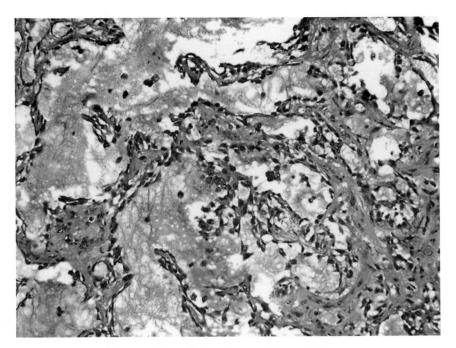

FIG. 5.14. Urothelial carcinoma with myxoid stroma.

In these cases, as mentioned earlier, diagnosis of invasion should rely on the characteristics of the invading epithelium.

Histologic Patterns of Lamina Propria Invasion

Lamina propria invasive tumors may be classified from their morphologic perspective according to several patterns (22) (Figs. 5.15, 5.16). Awareness of these patterns may be important to the surgical pathologist in order to focus on particular areas of the tumor while assessing for invasion, thus facilitating its recognition, even when it is extremely focal. Not all patterns are associated with clinical significance:

1. CIS with microinvasion: CIS may be associated with microinvasion (defined as invasion within superficial lamina propria no greater than 2 mm) (22,23) (Fig. 5.17). Invasion is histologically subtle, compounded by the fact that it is clinically not suspected and the obvious histologic focus is on the surface abnormality. Invasion may be in the form of single cells, clusters, or cords of cells or small nests of cells within the lamina propria. The stroma usually shows an inflammatory or desmoplastic reaction, or occasionally shows nests of tumor cells surrounded by retraction.

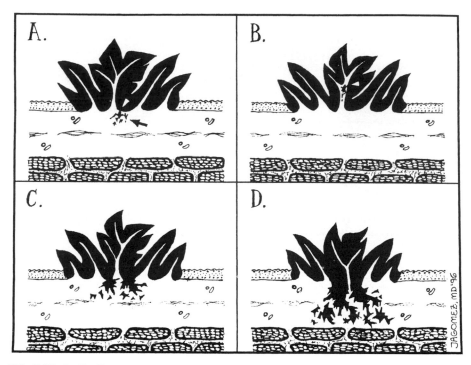

FIG. 5.15. A: Papillary urothelial carcinoma with microinvasion. **B:** Papillary urothelial carcinoma with invasion into stalk. **C:** Papillary urothelial carcinoma with lamina propria invasion (up to muscularis mucosae). **D:** Papillary urothelial carcinoma with lamina propria invasion (beyond the muscularis mucosae). (From Amin MB, Gomez JA, Young RH. Urothelial transitional cell carcinoma with endophytic growth patterns: a discussion of patterns of invasion and problems associated with assessment of invasion in 18 cases. *Am J Surg Pathol* 1997;21:1057–1068, with permission.)

2. Papillary urothelial carcinoma with microinvasion (Fig. 5.18): Microinvasion (less than 2 mm) of papillary tumors can be similarly defined as in cases with CIS and should be mentioned in the diagnosis to document minimal, focal, or early invasion.
3. Papillary urothelial carcinoma with invasion into stalk (Fig. 5.19): Very rarely, papillary urothelial carcinomas invade into the stalk of a tumor (22,24). Appreciation of this pattern requires optimal orientation of the entire or large parts of the papillary tumor, which may not always be the case, especially in TURBT specimens.
4. Well-established invasion into underlying lamina propria: In the overwhelming majority of cases, invasion is seen at the base of the papillary neoplasm (Fig. 5.7). With respect to the muscularis mucosae layer within the lamina propria, invasive tumors may be classified as follows:
   • Invasive up to the muscularis mucosae (Fig. 5.20).

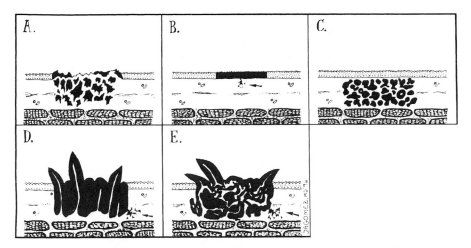

FIG. 5.16. A: Carcinoma in situ (CIS) with lamina propria invasion (beyond the muscularis mucosae). **B:** CIS with microinvasion. **C:** Urothelial carcinoma (nested variant). **D:** Papillary urothelial carcinoma with broad-front endophytic growth pattern and invasion. **E:** Papillary urothelial carcinoma with inverted papilloma-like growth pattern and invasion. (From Amin MB, Gomez JA, Young RH. Urothelial transitional cell carcinoma with endophytic growth patterns: a discussion of patterns of invasion and problems associated with assessment of invasion in 18 cases. *Am J Surg Pathol* 1997;21:1057–1068, with permission.)

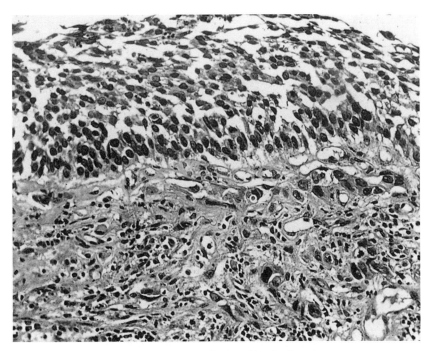

FIG. 5.17. Carcinoma in situ with microinvasion.

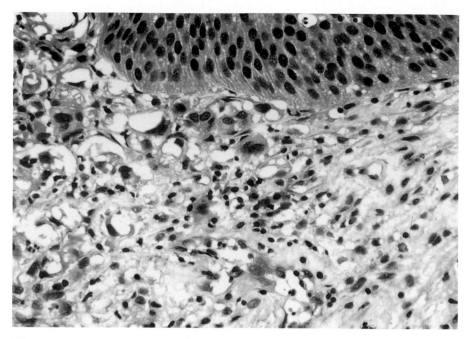

FIG. 5.18. Microinvasive individual infiltrating cells of urothelial carcinoma within high-grade papillary urothelial carcinoma.

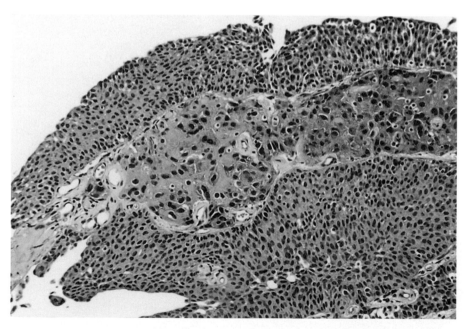

FIG. 5.19. Infiltrating carcinoma within stalk of papillary urothelial carcinoma. Note paradoxical differentiation where infiltrating component has more abundant cytoplasm than noninvasive component.

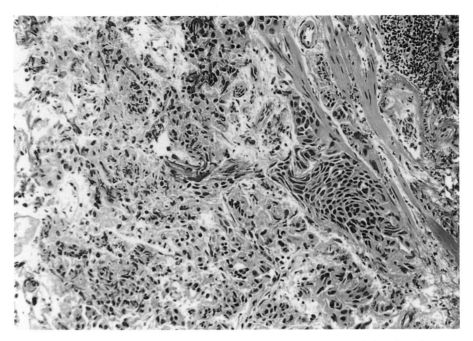

FIG. 5.20. Infiltrating high-grade urothelial carcinoma invading small muscle bundles of muscularis mucosae.

- Invasive beyond the muscularis mucosae, but not in the muscularis propria.
- Lamina propria invasion not further specified (no muscularis mucosae present). This categorization may have clinical implications, as presented later.
5. Urothelial carcinoma with endophytic or broad-front growth pattern (efigs 238, 277, 399–414) (see Chapter 4).

Problems and Pitfalls in the Diagnosis of T1 Invasion

Diagnosis of lamina propria invasion is often difficult, and the problem is well exemplified in the data from the French Association of Urology Cancer Committee study (10), which revealed that seven experienced pathologists could agree on lamina propria invasion in only 61% of cases after three assessments. In 10% of cases, no consensus was achieved despite four evaluations. In another study by Abel and colleagues (11), 15% of lesions initially diagnosed as T1 were downstaged to Ta and 22% of urothelial carcinomas diagnosed with muscle invasion were downstaged to T1 or Ta by a "dedicated" pathologist. To improve the concordance rates among pathologists, it is imperative to be aware of and understand the possible pitfalls in the diagnosis of lamina propria invasion (Table 5.2). The most common ones follow:

1. Tangential sectioning and poor orientation: Transurethral resections of bladder tumor specimens are excised in a piecemeal fashion, rendering fragmented specimens that are usually poorly oriented. Furthermore, because of their complex architecture, papillary tumors are inevitably tangentially sectioned in multiple planes, resulting in isolated nests of tumor cells within connective tissue. Smooth, round, and regular contours favor tangential sectioning, whereas irregular, jagged nests with haphazard arrangement favors stromal invasion.

2. Thermal injury: Thermal injury or cautery artifact produces severely distorted morphology in TURBT specimens and is a frequent source of distress for the pathologist. Pathologists have no control over this problem, although deeper levels may occasionally display better preserved areas. When this is not helpful, the pathologist should express the inability to render a definitive diagnosis due to thermal effect. Occasionally, we have used the cytokeratin stain to accentuate the presence of infiltrating carcinoma amidst necrotic or poorly preserved tissue.

3. Obscuring inflammation: Papillary tumors may show variable, often brisk inflammation at the tumor-stromal interface, which may obscure isolated cells or nests of invasive tumor. If suspicion for tumor is high or if large atypical cells are present in the lamina propria, judicious use of cytokeratin immunostaining may be useful.

4. CIS involving von Brunn nests: Flat lesions, when they involve von Brunn nests, may mimic lamina propria invasion by the mere presence of high-grade cells within the lamina propria. This is especially problematic in prominent nests or in those that have been distorted by an inflammatory process.

5. Muscle invasion indeterminate for type of muscle: In cases of invasive tumor that is juxtaposed to muscle fibers but due to obscuring factors (i.e., inflammation, tangential sectioning, cautery artifact, strong desmoplastic

TABLE 5.2. *Pitfalls in the diagnosis of lamina propria invasion by urothelial carcinoma*

Tangential sectioning
Thermal artifact
Obscuring inflammation
Carcinoma in situ involving von Brunn nests
Invasion into muscle, indeterminate for type of muscle (muscularis mucosae vs. muscularis propria)
Invasion into adipose tissue within lamina propria (overdiagnosis of extravesical invasion)
Deceptively bland urothelial carcinomas
  • Microcystic variant of urothelial carcinoma (invasive)
  • Broad front or inverted growth, raising the question of invasion
  • Nested variant of urothelial carcinoma (invasive)
Overdiagnosis of vascular invasion

response, or poor orientation) or when the caliber of the muscle bundles is such that it is difficult to distinguish between hypertrophic muscularis mucosae or muscularis propria bundles, the pathologist is unable to determine whether the muscle involved belongs to the muscularis mucosae or the muscularis propria (Fig. 5.21). It is recommended that, when faced with this situation, pathologists should clearly state their uncertainty in establishing the depth of invasion rather than commit to a particular type of muscle involvement—muscularis mucosae (T1) or muscularis propria (T2). This distinction is critical, in that muscularis propria invasion is currently regarded as the crossroads between conservative management and aggressive therapy.

6. Invasion into fat does not indicate extravesical spread: Fat may be normally present in the lamina propria; therefore, tumor invasive into fat should not automatically equate to involvement of perivesical fat (19).

7. Deceptively bland variants of urothelial carcinomas: When limited to the lamina propria, deceptively bland patterns of invasive urothelial carcinoma may make the recognition of T1 disease extremely difficult (see Chapter 6). For example, microcystic urothelial carcinoma (25) can easily mimic cystitis cystica, and the "nested" pattern may be easily confused with von Brunn

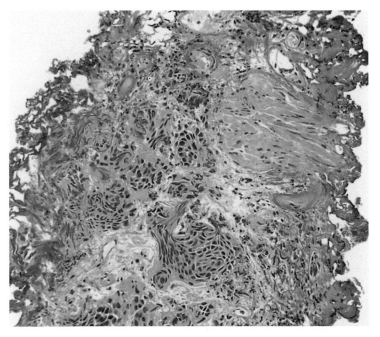

FIG. 5.21. Urothelial carcinoma invasive into muscle, indeterminate of muscle type (muscularis mucosae or muscularis propria). Cautery artifact and limited specimen precludes a definitive diagnosis.

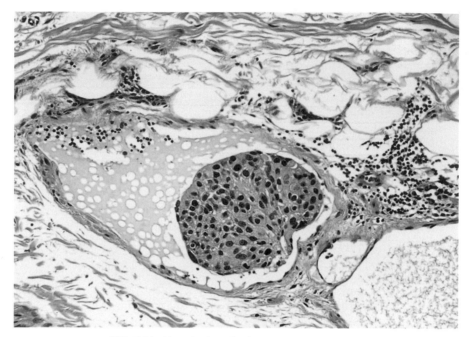

FIG. 5.22. Vascular invasion by urothelial carcinoma.

nests (26) (see Chapter 1). Attention should be paid to general features useful in assessing invasion, such as cytologic atypia, infiltrative architecture, desmoplasia, and architectural complexity, especially because they may appear subtle in superficial biopsies.

8. Overdiagnosis of vascular invasion: As discussed earlier, a peculiar stromal retraction artifact in lamina propria invasive tumors may mimic vascular

TABLE 5.3. *Criteria and pitfalls for vascular–lymphatic invasion in urothelial neoplasms*

Criteria for vascular–lymphatic invasion
  Presence of unequivocal endothelial lining
  Nests attached to wall of lumen containing blood constituents (red blood cells, inflammatory cells, or thrombus)
  Nests attached to and conforming to the shape of the vessel
  Peritumoral location of vascular invasion (intratumoral invasion not diagnostic by itself)
  Tumor cells in the space near large artery or vein (vascular route)
  Immunohistochemical confirmation (factor VIII or CD31)
Pitfalls in recognition of vascular–lymphatic invasion (efig 570)
  Pitfall in recognition of endothelial and venular spaces
    Retraction of stroma (particularly conspicuous in micropapillary tumors)
  Pitfall in recognition of large vessel invasion
    Carryover due to fragmentation of neoplasm

Adapted from Jiminez RE, Keane TE, Hardy HT, et al. pT$_1$ Urothelial carcinoma of the bladder: criteria for diagnosis, pitfalls, and clinical implications. *Adv Anat Pathol* 2000;7:13–25, with permission.

invasion. Caution is hence warranted and strict criteria should be used (Fig. 5.22) (efigs 529-537) (Table 5.3).

SUBSTAGING OF T1 DISEASE

Attempts have been made to identify prognostic factors within the category of T1 tumors. Toward this end, several studies have evaluated the issue of substaging T1 urothelial carcinomas (14,27–28), with most using the muscularis mucosae as an anatomic landmark to assess the depth of invasion (tumors above or into muscularis mucosae are T1a; tumors invasive below are T1b). In the absence of muscularis mucosae (muscularis mucosae is seen in 18% to 83% of TURBT specimens only), large vessels have been used as a substitute for muscularis mucosae to designate T1a versus T1b disease. Others have used the depth of invasion in millimeters from the basement membrane (29).

The aggregate data of many studies indicate that deep lamina propria invasion, whether assessed by the relation of the tumor to the muscularis mucosae or by direct micrometric measurement, identifies a subset of patients with T1 disease with a more adverse prognosis (14). Tumors invading beyond the muscularis mucosae tend to behave like muscularis propria invasive (T2) tumors.

The 1998 WHO/ISUP Consensus Conference Committee as well as the WHO(2003)/ISUP classification have recognized and encouraged the need to express some assessment of the degree or extent of invasion in the pathology report. At this point, however, it is thought that substaging of T1 tumors should not be universally adopted because there is no consistently applicable and reproducible method (30).

Muscularis Propria (Detrusor Muscle) Invasive Tumors

Urothelial cancers invading between thick distinct fascicles of muscle bundles of detrusor muscle characterize T2 urothelial cancer (Figs. 5.23–5.26) (efigs 538–570). Muscle invasive carcinoma may or may not elicit a desmoplastic stromal response. In the T staging system, T2 tumors are divided into those invading the inner half (T2a) and those invading the outer half (T2b). Because TURBT specimens lack orientation with respect to bladder anatomy, substaging of T2 disease should be performed in cystectomy specimens alone. Also, because there is often abundant adipose tissue between detrusor muscle bundles, the presence of tumor in adipose tissue in a TURBT specimen does not necessarily equate to perivesical fat involvement. Hence, pathologic staging in TURBT specimens is limited to whether the tumor is Ta, T1, or T2. The distinction between T2a, T2b, and pT3 cancer is, hence, performed in cystectomy specimens alone. Because the junction between the muscularis propria layer and perivesical fat is not well demarcated while determining the status of a tumor as T2 or T3, an imaginary line may be drawn at low power to demarcate the boundary between the bladder wall in a cystectomy specimen and perivesical tissue.

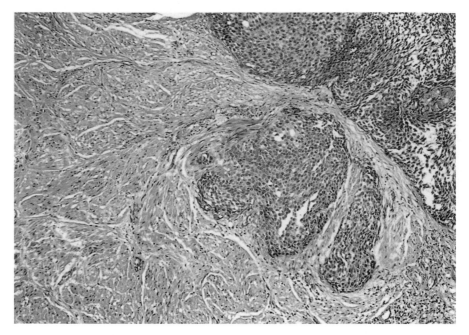

FIG. 5.23. Muscularis propria (detrusor muscle) invasion.

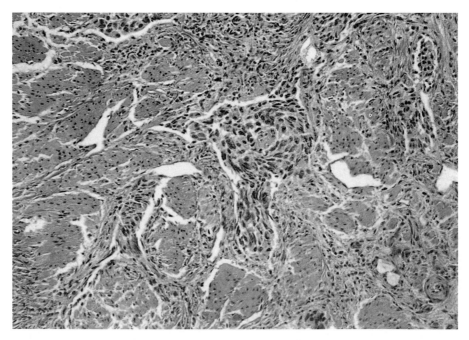

FIG. 5.24. Muscularis propria (detrusor muscle) invasion.

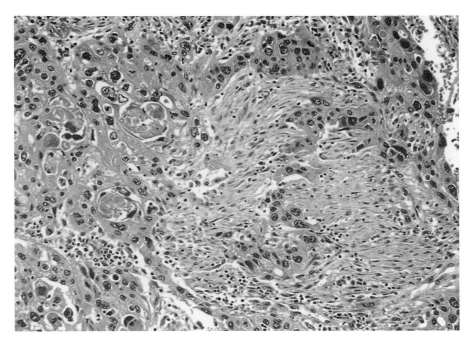

FIG. 5.25. Muscularis propria (detrusor muscle) invasion.

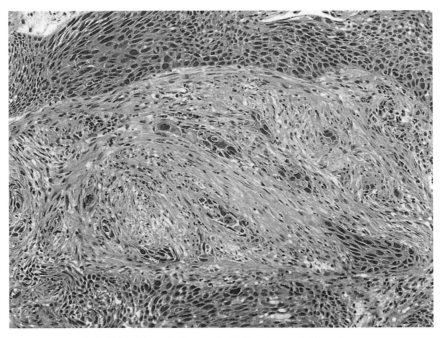

FIG. 5.26. Muscularis propria (detrusor muscle) invasion.

REFERENCES

1. Dalbagni G, Genega E, Hashibe M, et al. Cystectomy for bladder cancer: a contemporary series. *J Urol* 2001;165:1111–1116.
2. Logothetis CJ, Dexeus FH, Chong C, et al. Cisplatin, cyclophosphamide and doxorubicin chemotherapy for unresectable urothelial tumors: the M.D. Anderson experience. *J Urol* 1989;141:33–37.
3. Akdas A, Turkeri L. The impact of squamous metaplasia in transitional cell carcinoma of the bladder. *Int Urol Nephrol* 1991;23:333–336.
4. Larsen MP, Steinberg GD, Brendler CB, et al. Use of Ulex europaeus agglutinin I (UEAI) to distinguish vascular and "pseudovascular" invasion in transitional cell carcinoma of bladder with lamina propria invasion. *Mod Pathol* 1990;3:83–88.
5. Ramani P, Birch BR, Harland SJ, et al. Evaluation of endothelial markers in detecting blood and lymphatic channel invasion in pT1 transitional carcinoma of bladder. *Histopathology* 1991;19:551–554.
6. American Joint Commission on Cancer. *AJCC cancer staging manual*, 5th ed. New York: Lippincott–Raven, 1997:302.
7. Anderstrom C, Johansson S, Nilsson S. The significance of lamina propria invasion on the prognosis of patients with bladder tumors. *J Urol* 1980;124:23–26.
8. Williams JL, Hammonds JC, Saunders N. T1 bladder tumours. *Br J Urol* 1977;49:663–668.
9. Kiemeney LA, Witjes JA, Verbeek AL, et al. The clinical epidemiology of superficial bladder cancer. Dutch South-East Cooperative Urological Group. *Br J Cancer* 1993;67:806–812.
10. Lamina propria microinvasion of bladder tumors, incidence on stage allocation (pTa vs pT1): recommended approach. Pathologists of the French Association of Urology Cancer Committee. *World J Urol* 1993;11:161–164.
11. Abel PD, Henderson D, Bennett MK, et al. Differing interpretations by pathologists of the pT category and grade of transitional cell cancer of the bladder. *Br J Urol* 1988;62:339–342.
12. Angulo JC, Lopez JI, Grignon DJ, et al. Muscularis mucosa differentiates two populations with different prognosis in stage T1 bladder cancer. *Urology* 1995;45:47–53.
13. Sarkis AS, Dalbagni G, Cordon-Cardo C, et al. Nuclear overexpression of p53 protein in transitional cell bladder carcinoma: a marker for disease progression. *J Natl Cancer Inst* 1993;85:53–59.
14. Jimenez RE, Keane TE, Hardy HT, et al. pT$_1$ Urothelial carcinoma of the bladder: criteria for diagnosis, pitfalls, and clinical implications. *Adv Anat Pathol* 2000;7:13–25.
15. Dixon JS, Gosling JA. Histology and fine structure of the muscularis mucosae of the human urinary bladder. *J Anat* 1983;136:265–271.
16. Ro JY, Ayala AG, el-Naggar A. Muscularis mucosa of urinary bladder. Importance for staging and treatment. *Am J Surg Pathol* 1987;11:668–673.
17. Keep JC, Piehl M, Miller A, et al. Invasive carcinomas of the urinary bladder. Evaluation of tunica muscularis mucosae involvement. *Am J Clin Pathol* 1989;91:575–579.
18. Platz CE, Cohen MB, Jones MP, et al. Is microstaging of early invasive cancer of the urinary bladder possible or useful? *Mod Pathol* 1996;9:1035–1039.
19. Philip AT, Amin MB, Tamboli P, et al. Intravesical adipose tissue. A quantitative study of its presence and location with implications for therapy and prognosis. *Am J Surg Pathol* 2000;24:1286–1290.
20. Amin MB, Murphy WM, Reuter VE, et al. Controversies in the pathology of transitional cell carcinoma of the urinary bladder. Part II. In: Rosen PP, Fechner RE, eds. *Reviews of pathology*. Chicago: ASCP Press, 1997:72–100.
21. Young RH, Wick MR. Transitional cell carcinoma of the urinary bladder with pseudosarcomatous stroma. *Am J Clin Pathol* 1988;90:216–219.
22. Amin MB, Gomez JA, Young RH. Urothelial transitional cell carcinoma with endophytic growth patterns: a discussion of patterns of invasion and problems associated with assessment of invasion in 18 cases. *Am J Surg Pathol* 1997;21:1057–1068.
23. McKenney J, Gomez JA, Desai S, et al. Morphologic expressions of urothelial carcinoma in situ. A detailed evaluation of its histologic patterns with emphasis on carcinoma in situ with microinvasion. *Am J Surg Pathol* 2001;25:356–362.
24. Pagano F, PegoraroV, Prayer-Galetti T, et al. Prognosis of bladder cancer-II. The fate of patients with T1b transitional cell bladder cancer. *Eur Urol* 1987;13:305–309.
25. Young RH, Zukerberg LR. Microcystic transitional cell carcinomas of the urinary bladder. A report of four cases. *Am J Clin Pathol* 1991;96:635–639.
26. Drew PA, Furman J, Civantos F, et al. The nested variant of transitional cell carcinoma: an aggressive neoplasm with innocuous histology. *Mod Pathol* 1996;9:989–994.

27. Younes M, Sussman J, True LD. The usefulness of the level of the muscularis mucosae in the staging of invasive transitional cell carcinoma of the urinary bladder. *Cancer* 1990;66:543–548.
28. Holmang S, Hedelin H, Anderstrom C, et al. The importance of the depth of invasion in stage T1 bladder carcinoma: a prospective cohort study. *J Urol* 1997;157:800–803; discussion 804.
29. Cheng L, Weaver AL, Neumann RM, et al. Substaging of T1 bladder carcinoma based on the depth of invasion: a new proposal. *Cancer* 1999;86:1035–1043.
30. Epstein JI, Amin MB, Reuter VR, et al. The World Health Organization/International Society of Urological Pathology consensus classification of urothelial (transitional cell) neoplasms of the urinary bladder. Bladder Consensus Conference Committee. *Am J Surg Pathol* 1998;22:1435–1448.

6

Histologic Variants of Urothelial Carcinoma

With increasing experience with urothelial carcinomas at the light microscopic level, the spectrum of microscopic forms of urothelial carcinoma has been expanded to include several unusual histologic variants (1,2). The term *variant* is used to describe a distinctively different histomorphologic phenotype of a certain type of neoplasm. By definition, they arise from the surface urothelium. The recognition of histologic variants is important because (a) some types may be associated with a different clinical outcome, (b) some may have a different therapeutic approach, or (c) awareness of the unusual pattern may be critical in avoiding diagnostic misinterpretations. We generally recommend following two general rules when dealing with histologic variants. First, the variant histology should be documented in the pathology reports because metastatic tumors usually continue to exhibit the distinctive histologic pattern and knowledge of the variant histology facilitates association of the metastasis to the primary tumor. Second, because the pattern of the neoplasm deviates from the conventional form, the possibility that this "unusual" morphology represents a metastasis should be considered and ruled out.

DECEPTIVELY BENIGN VARIANTS OF UROTHELIAL CARCINOMA

Some urothelial carcinomas have histologic variants that mimic nonneoplastic conditions such as cystitis cystica, von Brunn nests, nephrogenic adenoma, and inverted papilloma (3–6). Awareness of these variants is important because limited sampling, particularly in cystoscopic biopsy specimens, could lead to an underdiagnosis of malignancy (3–6).

Nested Variant of Urothelial Carcinoma

This variant has distinct patterns in the superficial and deep portions. In superficial biopsy samples and transurethral resectates, the superficial component appears as discrete nests, occasionally with tubules (3–9) (Figs. 6.1–6.12) (efigs 571–599). The nests are tightly packed, often confluent and haphazardly arranged with little or no intervening stroma. Most nests have a relatively bland cytologic appearance, but at least some have more pleomorphic nuclei and large nucleoli. Overlying papillary carcinoma or recognizable flat in situ disease is most often not present (10). The architectural complexity, confluence, and anastomosis between the nests are features that are particularly helpful in distinguishing carcinoma from von Brunn nests or other benign conditions. In the deeper portion, the neoplasm usually shows greater cytologic atypia and an irregular infiltrative pattern. These tumors are frequently muscle invasive and, despite their innocuous histology, are paradoxically associated with aggressive clinical outcome. Even with therapy, 70% of patients with adequate follow-up died within 4 to 40 months of diagnosis (3–9). Another differential diagnostic consideration is nephrogenic adenoma (metaplasia) with a more solid appearance (6). The problem is compounded when the nephrogenic adenoma has an "infiltrative" growth at the base. The marked variation or occasional large nests, nuclear atypia in deeper aspects, stromal reaction, and muscularis propria invasion argue for a nested carcinoma diagnosis. Nephrogenic adenoma may show other coexisting patterns (tubules, papillary, signet ring, cystic) and often con-

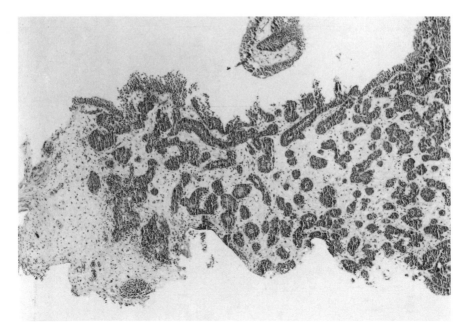

FIG. 6.1. Nested variant of urothelial carcinoma with irregular proliferation of nests within edematous lamina propria.

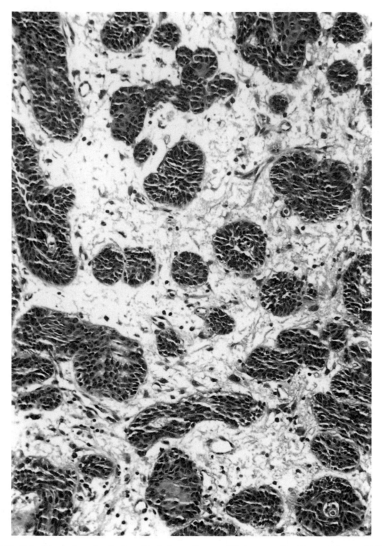

FIG. 6.2. Nested variant of urothelial carcinoma (high magnification of Figure 6.1).

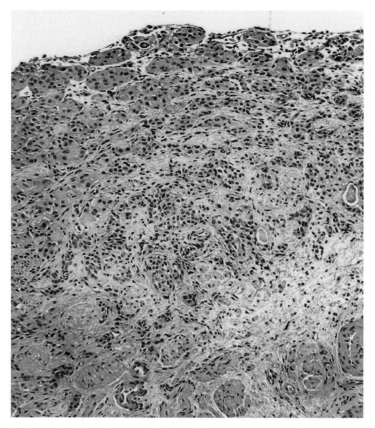

FIG. 6.3. Nested variant of urothelial carcinoma with extension of nests into muscularis mucosae.

tains stroma that is edematous and inflamed. Paraganglioma of the bladder and carcinoid tumor are other entities in the bladder that have overlapping features with the nested variant, but they also have other characteristics sufficient to warrant appropriate recognition. From a pathologist's perspective, the nested variant should appropriately be recognized as a malignant process; this pattern is particularly challenging in superficial biopsies.

Urothelial Carcinoma with Small Tubules

Some urothelial carcinomas may have a prominent component of small-sized to medium-sized, round to elongated tubules that may be misdiagnosed as

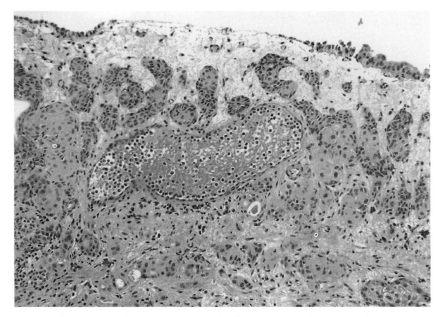

FIG. 6.4. Nested variant of urothelial carcinoma. The nests are too small and crowded to represent von Brunn nests.

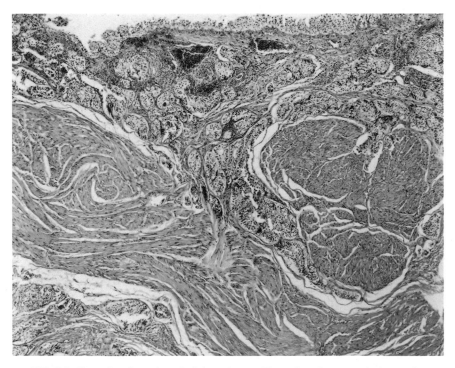

FIG. 6.5. Nested variant of urothelial carcinoma. Tumor invades muscularis propria.

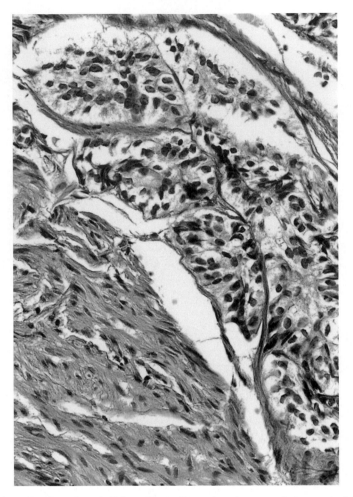

FIG. 6.6. Nested variant of urothelial carcinoma. Tumor invades muscularis propria (higher magnification of Figure 6.5).

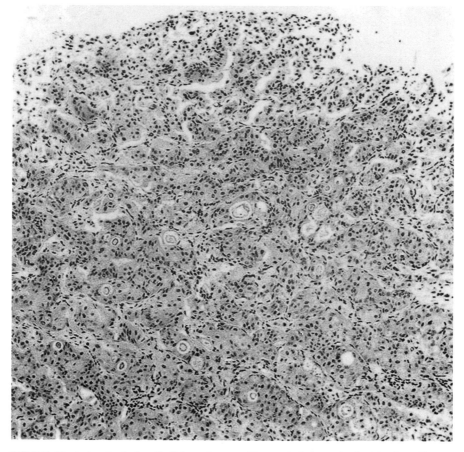

FIG. 6.7. Nested variant of urothelial carcinoma with crowded almost back-to-back proliferation of small nests.

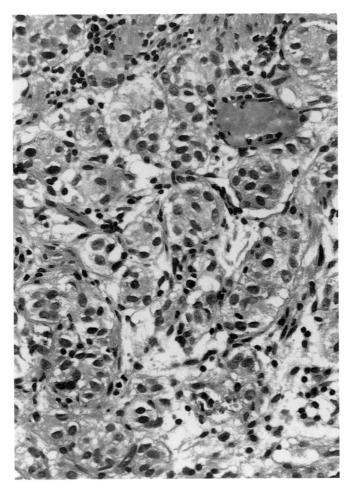

FIG. 6.8. Nested variant of urothelial carcinoma (higher magnification of Figure 6.7).

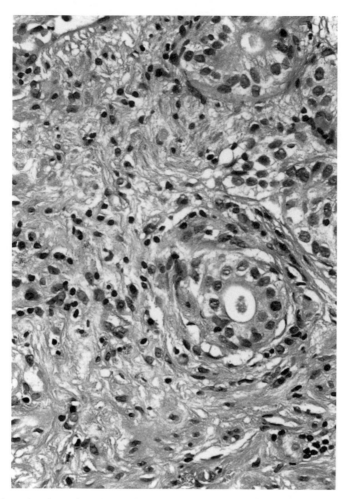

FIG. 6.9. Nested variant of urothelial carcinoma with focal tubule formation (higher magnification of Figure 6.7).

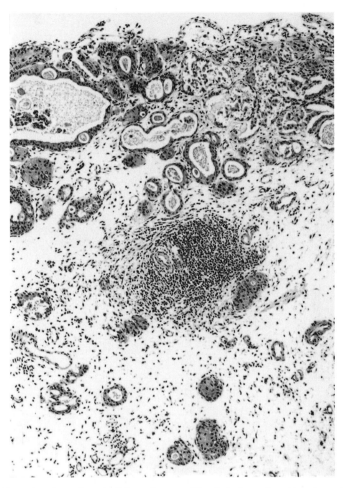

FIG. 6.10. Nested variant of urothelial carcinoma with tubule formation. Note irregular proliferation of nests and tubules in inflamed, edematous stroma.

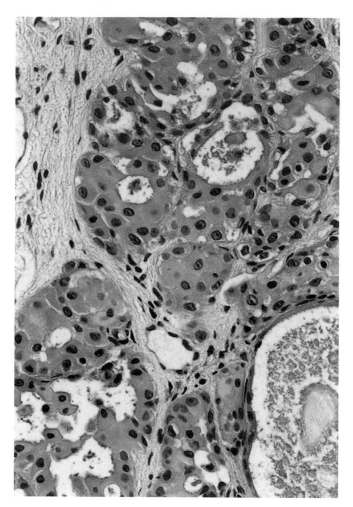

FIG. 6.11. Nested variant of urothelial carcinoma with moderate atypia (higher magnification of Figure 6.10).

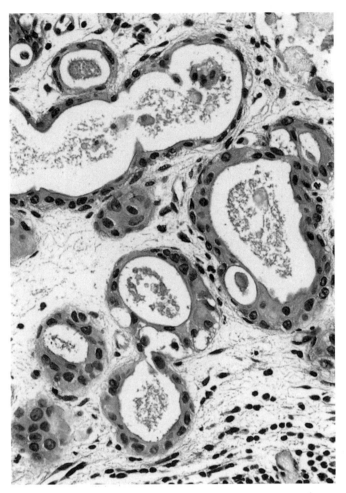

FIG. 6.12. Nested variant of urothelial carcinoma with tubule formation (higher magnification of Figure 6.10).

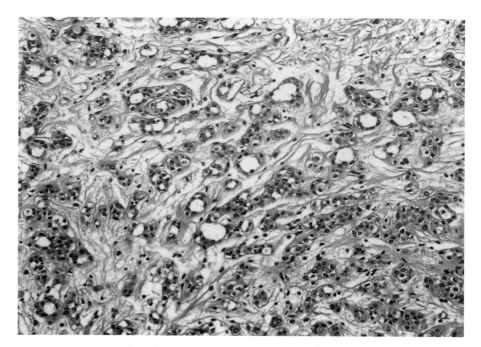

FIG. 6.13. Urothelial carcinoma with tubular differentiation.

nephrogenic adenoma (metaplasia) or cystitis glandularis (5,11) (Fig. 6.13) (efigs 600–602). The tubules, however, are lined by urothelial cells in contrast to the cuboidal, columnar, or occasionally flattened cells that line the tubules of nephrogenic adenoma. The cytologic features are invariably low grade, but the recognition of carcinoma is based on diffusely infiltrative architecture, considerable variation of tubular shape with haphazard organization, and the frequent presence of muscle invasion. The biologic significance of this pattern is uncertain, but some of these cases occur in conjunction with the nested pattern and may result in an aggressive behavior.

Microcystic Urothelial Carcinoma

This is yet another deceptively benign form of urothelial carcinoma and is exemplified by the formation of numerous microcysts, which may lead to the misdiagnosis of cystitis cystica upon superficial examination or in limited biopsy specimens (12–14) (Fig. 6.14) (efigs 603, 604). The pattern is characterized by prominent widespread cystic change of variable size within nests of urothelial carcinoma or within urothelial carcinoma with glandular differentiation. The cysts are round to oval, 1 to 2 mm in size, and contain secretions that

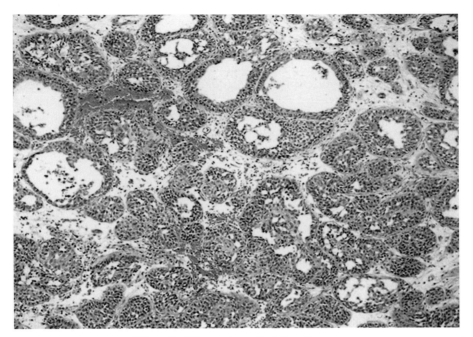

FIG. 6.14. Microcystic urothelial carcinoma.

may be targetoid. The cyst lining is most commonly urothelial and is usually focally glandular; larger cysts may possess a flattened epithelium or a denuded lining. Cytologic blandness is present by definition, and the most critical feature in distinguishing this carcinoma type from benign conditions is the variation, often dramatic, in size and shape of the epithelial formations and the relatively haphazard infiltrative growth into the wall of the urinary bladder. There is no striking biologic significance associated with this pattern, except that it represents a potentially serious diagnostic pitfall, particularly in limited samples (12,14). Once again, the nested, small tubule, and cystic variants may coexist in the same lesion (5).

Inverted Papilloma-like Growth Pattern of Urothelial Carcinoma

This form of urothelial carcinoma is associated with two diagnostic concerns: (a) distinction from inverted papilloma (see Chapter 4) and (b) difficulty in assessing invasion (see Chapter 5) (15,16). Distinction from the inverted papilloma requires attention to the architectural and cytologic features of the lesion. Urothelial carcinomas with inverted growth usually have thicker columns, with irregularity in width of the columns or transition of cords and columns into more solid areas (efigs 277–283, 399–414). The characteristic orderly maturation, spindling, and peripheral palisading seen in inverted papilloma are generally absent or inconspicuous in urothelial carcinomas with inverted growth. Unequivocal stromal invasion into the lamina propria or muscularis propria rules out the diagnosis of inverted papilloma, as does the presence of appreciable exophytic papillary architecture. Furthermore, cytologic atypia is an important feature for the diagnosis of carcinoma; thus, carcinomas with inverted growth, like their exophytic counterparts, may be classified as low grade or high grade. Inverted urothelial carcinoma may or may not be associated with destructive invasion (see Chapter 5 for criteria for invasion).

MICROPAPILLARY VARIANT OF UROTHELIAL CARCINOMA

This histologic variant of urothelial carcinoma has a micropapillary architecture that is reminiscent of the papillary configuration seen in ovarian papillary serous tumors (17–21). This rare histologic variant comprises 0.6% to 1% of urothelial carcinomas and shows a definite male predominance (male-to-female ratio 5:1) that is higher than in conventional urothelial carcinoma (3:1). More than 95% of these tumors are muscle invasive at the time of presentation. Histologically, the micropapillary component of these tumors may be encountered in

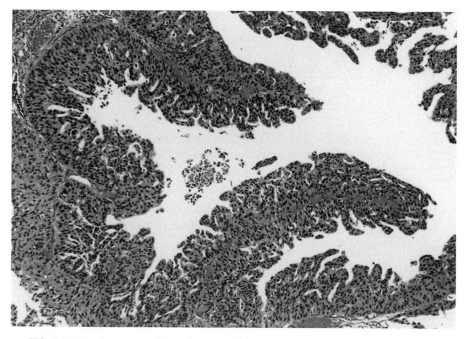

FIG. 6.15. Noninvasive and invasive urothelial carcinoma with micropapillary features.

(a) the noninvasive component, (b) the invasive component, and (c) metastasis. This pattern may be focal, extensive (greater than 90%), or exclusive. Urothelial carcinoma in situ (urothelial CIS) is demonstrable in greater than 50% of the cases and concurrent glandular differentiation is known to occur. Five histologic features of the micropapillary component are noteworthy. First, micropapillary carcinoma has two distinct patterns: on the surface it forms slender, delicate filiform processes, rarely with a fibrovascular core (Figs. 6.15–6.17) (efigs 605–610). When cut in cross sections, these papillae appear as glomeruloid bodies. In the invasive component and in all metastatic sites, the tumor cells are arranged in small tight nests or balls (Figs. 6.18–6.20) (Color Plate 5) (efigs 611–630). Second, psammoma bodies, a feature of ovarian papillary serous neoplasia, are exquisitely rare in micropapillary carcinoma. Third, the tumor cells in the invasive and metastatic components are aggregated in lacunae, which mimic vascular invasion. This feature is intriguing and extremely characteristic of invasive micropapillary carcinoma. The spaces may be lined focally by flattened spindled cells or may be devoid of any lining. In most instances, there is no host response to the tumor cells that merely seem to reside in hollow spaces at various random intervals within the tumor (17). This pattern of lacunae containing neoplastic cells is also seen in the metastatic sites. Awareness that lacunae of micropapillary urothelial carcinoma may mimic vascular invasion is important

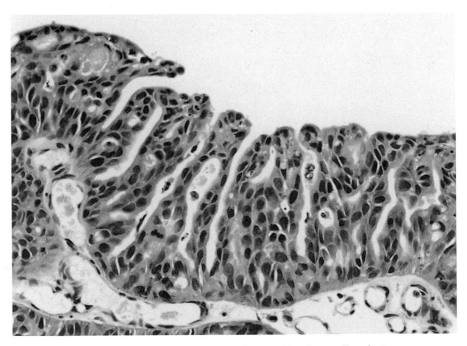

FIG. 6.16. Noninvasive urothelial carcinoma with micropapillary features.

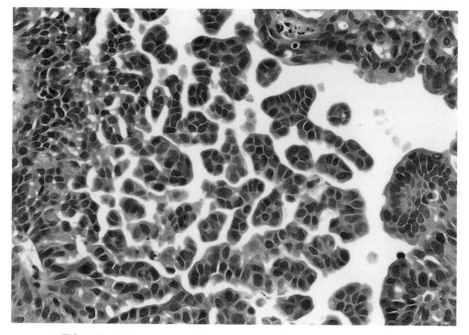

FIG. 6.17. Noninvasive urothelial carcinoma with micropapillary features.

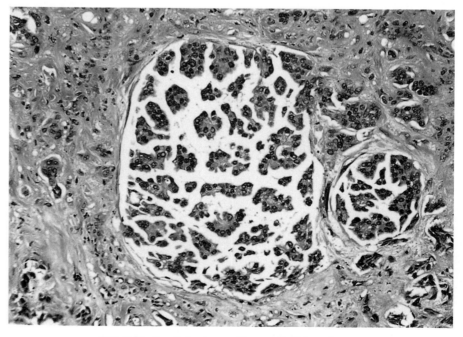

FIG. 6.18. Invasive micropapillary urothelial carcinoma.

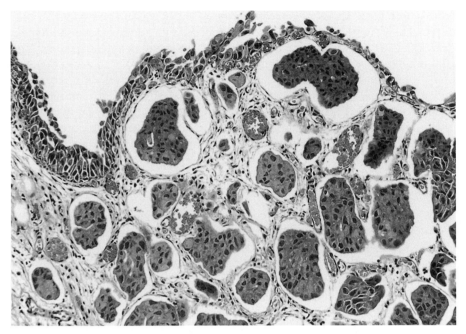

FIG. 6.19. Invasive micropapillary carcinoma beneath urothelium, mimicking vascular invasion.

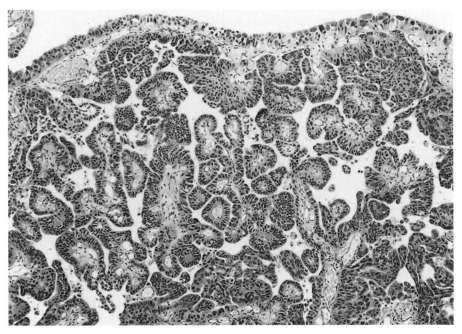

FIG. 6.20. Invasive micropapillary carcinoma beneath urothelium.

so that one does not overdiagnose the presence of vascular invasion. Fourth, micropapillary carcinoma always demonstrates a high nuclear grade (high grade by WHO/ISUP classification), although some areas within a neoplasm may parallel low-grade urothelial carcinoma. Fifth, most reported cases with micropapillary carcinoma show at least focal unequivocal vascular invasion. Like urothelial carcinomas, the tumors are positive for CK7, CK20, and epithelial membrane antigen (22). Leu-M$_1$, CEA, and Ca antigen 125 may be focally positive, in keeping with glandular differentiation that may be concurrent.

There are several important reasons for recognizing the micropapillary variant of urothelial carcinoma:

1. These tumors are high grade and high stage and are almost always associated with vascular invasion.
2. Micropapillary carcinoma has a higher DNA index than conventional urothelial carcinoma (limited cases examined) (17), and, because metastatic sites of tumors with micropapillary histology are predominantly composed of micropapillary carcinoma, it is likely that this unique configuration of urothelial carcinoma connotes a more aggressive clone of neoplastic cells.
3. The presence of micropapillary histology in metastatic sites forces one to consider the possibility of urothelial carcinoma, especially if the micropapillary configuration is encountered in the peritoneum, abdominal lymph nodes, or mesentery of a male patient with an unknown primary or in a female patient with no apparent abnormality of the gynecologic tract (17–20). One of the authors (M.B.A.) has seen two cases presenting in supraclavicular lymph nodes of male patients.
4. The high association of micropapillary carcinoma with muscle invasive disease should make the pathologist look diligently for muscle invasion if it is not readily apparent. If the biopsy is superficial and lacks muscularis propria, a second biopsy should be considered.

LYMPHOEPITHELIOMA-LIKE CARCINOMA

Tumors with this histology are so termed because of their striking morphologic resemblance to the undifferentiated nasopharyngeal carcinoma or lymphoepithelioma (23,24) (Figs. 6.21–6.23) (efigs 631–646). The neoplastic cells are large and arranged in sheets, cords, or trabeculae with syncytia of cells containing vesicular nuclei, prominent nucleoli, and numerous mitoses (23–27). The sine qua non for the diagnosis of this histologic pattern of urothelial carcinoma is the presence of a prominent lymphoid infiltrate, although an admixture of other inflammatory cells including plasma cells and eosinophils is not uncommon. No association with Epstein-Barr virus has been found thus far (28). The tumors may occur in a pure form or the lymphoepithelioma-like histology may be predominant or focal. CIS may be present elsewhere in the bladder. The tumor cells are positive for cytokeratin, CK7, and CK8, and are rarely positive for

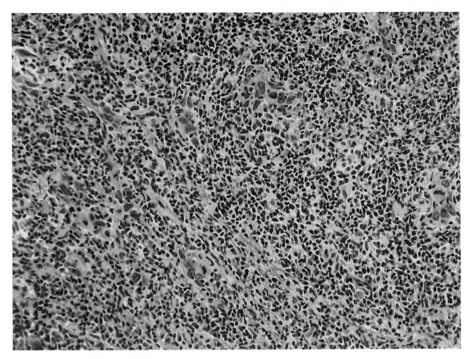

FIG. 6.21. Lymphoepithelioma-like carcinoma.

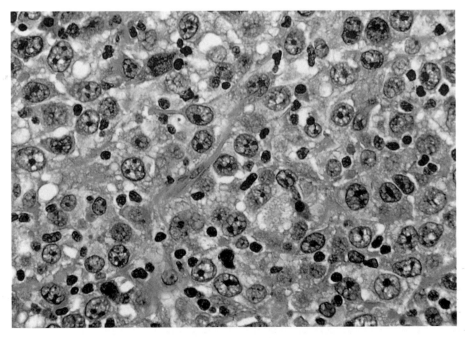

FIG. 6.22. Lymphoepithelioma-like carcinoma.

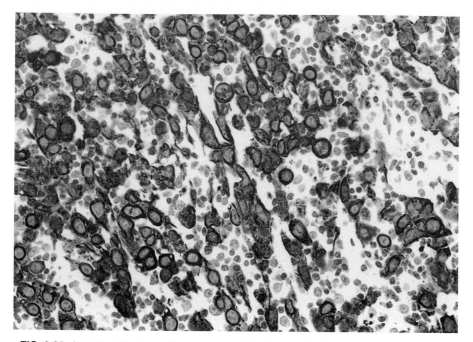

FIG. 6.23. Lymphoepithelioma-like carcinoma. Keratin stain highlights epithelial tumor cells.

CK20. Relatively few series and cases of this subtype of urothelial carcinoma have been reported, but the aggregate data suggest that when these tumors occur in a pure form they are more responsive to systemic chemotherapy, providing the potential to salvage bladder function (23–27). When mixed with conventional urothelial carcinoma, their outcome is similar to that for conventional urothelial carcinoma and depends on the stage of the associated conventional urothelial carcinoma. The differential diagnosis includes malignant lymphoma and, in limited and crushed biopsies, marked chronic cystitis (29). High-grade urothelial carcinoma of the usual type should not be termed lymphoepithelioma-like merely because of a brisk inflammatory infiltrate. The syncytial arrangement and typical cytology are essential for the diagnosis of lymphoepithelioma-like carcinoma which, as mentioned, in its purest form may be treated differently than the usual or conventional invasive carcinoma.

SARCOMATOID CARCINOMA (CARCINOSARCOMA)

Although rare, sarcomatoid carcinoma is more common than primary sarcoma of the urinary bladder. By definition, this is a biphasic tumor composed of a malignant spindle cell component and a malignant epithelial component (30–35) (Figs. 6.24–6.31) (Color Plate 6) (efigs 647–691). The spindle cell com-

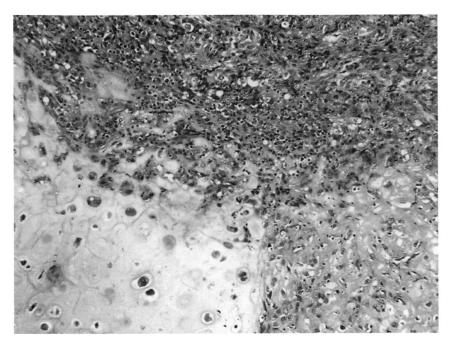

FIG. 6.24. Sarcomatoid carcinoma. Note malignant cartilage.

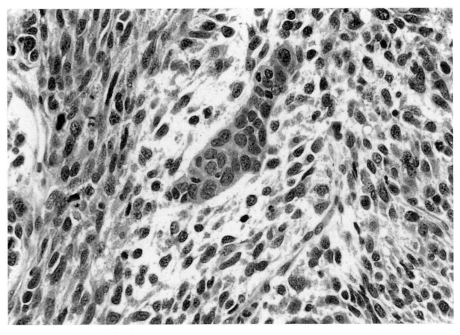

FIG. 6.25. Sarcomatoid carcinoma with nest of urothelial carcinoma surrounded by undifferentiated sarcomatoid component.

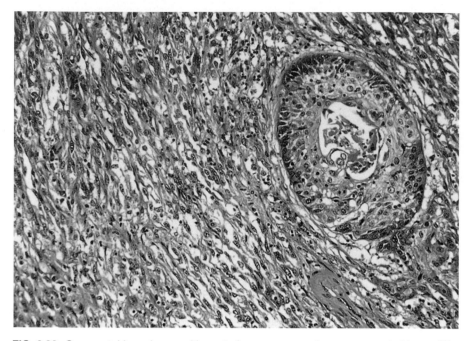

FIG. 6.26. Sarcomatoid carcinoma with nest of squamous carcinoma surrounded by undifferentiated sarcomatoid component.

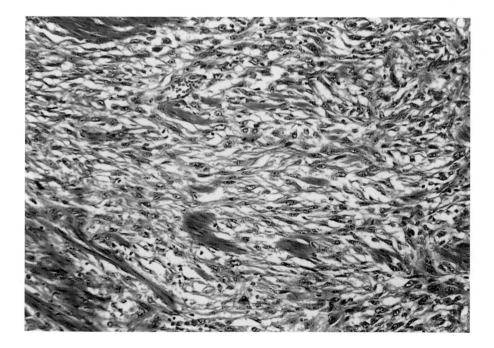

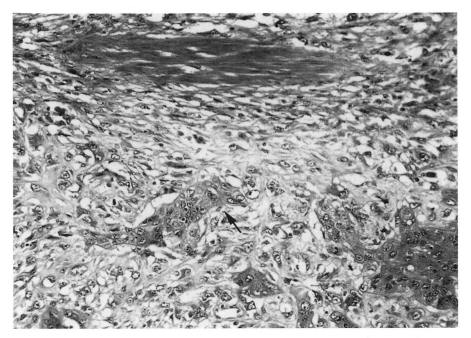

FIG. 6.28. Sarcomatoid carcinoma (higher magnification of Figure 6.27) showing focal nests of carcinoma (*arrow*).

ponent is usually high grade with nondescript architecture (often resembling malignant fibrous histiocytoma). The sarcomatoid areas may merge with foci of overlying CIS or with invasive urothelial carcinoma, squamous cell carcinoma, adenocarcinoma, or small cell carcinoma. Heterologous differentiation (carcinosarcoma) in the form of rhabdomyosarcomatous, osteosarcomatous, chondrosarcomatous, and the like may be present but to date has no prognostic significance. For the same reasons given in cases with focal glandular or squamous differentiation, the presence and relative amount of any mesenchymal elements should be mentioned in the pathology report. Grossly, many tumors present as polypoid masses. Almost all sarcomatoid carcinomas present at a high stage and have a poor prognosis (30–35). These tumors do not demonstrate a difference in survival when compared stage-for-stage with urothelial carcinoma (30–35). In the absence of an obvious invasive urothelial carcinoma or other epithelial dif-

---

FIG. 6.27. Sarcomatoid carcinoma mostly composed of undifferentiated malignant spindle cells. Tumor infiltrated muscularis propria.

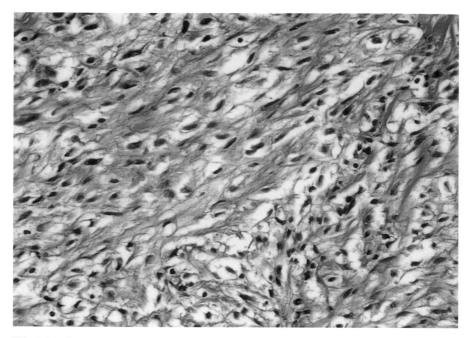

FIG. 6.29. Sarcomatoid carcinoma (higher magnification of Figure 6.27) showing focal areas where sarcomatoid component had relatively bland cytology.

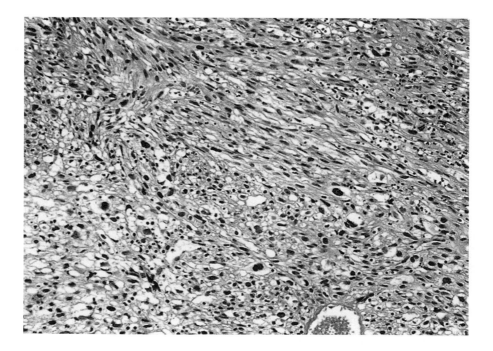

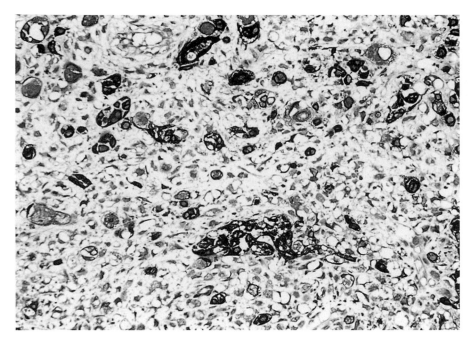

FIG. 6.31. Sarcomatoid carcinoma (higher magnification of Figure 6.30) with keratin positivity documenting epithelial differentiation.

ferentiation, the history of prior urothelial carcinoma, the coexistence of urothelial CIS, or strong cytokeratin immunoreactivity is helpful in making the diagnosis of sarcomatoid carcinoma over a primary sarcoma. The adjuvant therapy for sarcomatoid carcinoma tends to vary from institution to institution and may be different from therapy for a primary sarcoma. The epithelial elements are consistently positive for cytokeratin, but the reactivity in the malignant spindle cell component varies. The spindle cell component is consistently positive for vimentin and may express specific markers corresponding to specific mesenchymal differentiation if present. The cytologic atypia present in these lesions and the concurrent presence of neoplastic epithelial elements should exclude nonneoplastic lesions such as postoperative spindle cell nodule and inflammatory myofibroblastic tumors (36). A subset of sarcomatoid carcinomas have a markedly myxoid stroma that may result in some cases of sarcomatoid carcinoma ("myxoid and sclerosing sarcomatoid urothelial carcinoma") being diagnosed as inflammatory myofibroblastic tumors (34). The presence of a malignant epithelial component rules out the diagnosis of a primary sarcoma. Finally,

FIG. 6.30. Sarcomatoid carcinoma composed entirely of sarcomatous-appearing cells.

sarcomatoid carcinoma should be distinguished from the rare carcinoma with metaplastic, benign-appearing bone or cartilage in the stroma or from carcinoma associated with an unusual degenerative yet atypical appearing stromal reaction (pseudosarcomatous stromal reaction) (see pages 135–136) (37,38).

SMALL CELL CARCINOMA AND OTHER NEUROENDOCRINE TUMORS

The gross features of this tumor are not characteristic, and tumors may appear sessile, nodular, ulcerated, polypoid, or infiltrative. They are, however, usually very large and arise from all regions of the bladder, including in diverticula. Morphologically, this tumor is identical to small cell carcinoma of the lung with the notable exception that approximately half of the cases are admixed with urothelial carcinoma, squamous cell carcinoma, adenocarcinoma, sarcomatoid carcinoma, or a mixture of carcinomatous components (39–46) (Figs. 6.32, 6.33) (Color Plate 7) (efigs 692–704). In some cases of apparently pure small cell carcinoma, a urothelial CIS component may be present, confirming its association with urothelial carcinoma. The tumor histology is fairly characteristic on low power with a diffuse, patternless arrangement of round, blue hyperchromatic cells interspersed with areas of focal geographic necrosis. Organoid and trabecular arrangement is unusual but possible. The cells, approximately three times

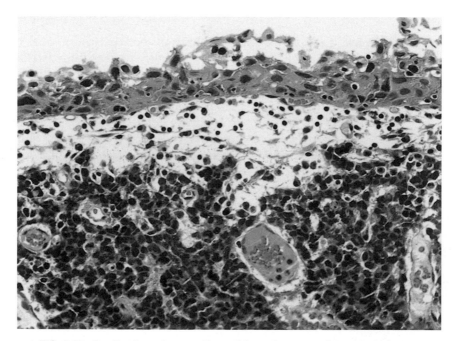

FIG. 6.32. Small cell carcinoma with overlying squamous cell carcinoma in situ.

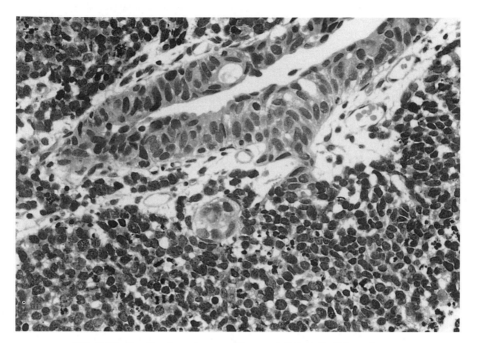

FIG. 6.33. Small cell carcinoma with associated urothelial carcinoma.

the size of lymphocytes, have granular chromatin, inconspicuous nucleoli, and frequent mitoses. The cytoplasm is typically scant with molding of nuclei. Rarely, large monstrous or multinucleated cells may be present. One case with rhabdomyosarcomatous differentiation is reported (47). The tumors are almost without exception widely invasive and involve muscle; invasion into perivesical fat is not uncommon. Small cell carcinoma of the urinary bladder has been associated with paraneoplastic syndromes, high stage at presentation, and frequent disseminated metastases, including metastases to viscera, bone, and brain (39–46). The overall 5-year cancer-free survival is 29% and correlates with stage of disease. An important reason for its recognition is the apparent response to newer chemotherapy protocols (mostly cisplatin-based), which, in combination with surgical resection, have shown encouraging results; reports of long-term survivors are available (39,48–50). Given its propensity for early systemic dissemination, some institutions opt for systemic chemotherapy before surgical resection (neoadjuvant chemotherapy). The diagnosis of small cell carcinoma, therefore, has prognostic and therapeutic implications.

Although a wide range of immunohistochemical antibodies has been reported in small cell carcinoma of the bladder, from a diagnostic perspective, chromogranin, synaptophysin, and cytokeratin (often dotlike positivity) are usually sufficient. Thyroid transcription factor 1 (TTF-1) has been shown to be positive in some primary bladder small cell carcinomas and in a significantly large number of pulmonary small cell carcinomas (51). Ultrastructural studies have demonstrated dense core granules (150 to 250 mm) in all cases studied with tonofilaments, dendrite-like processes, and variably intercellular lumina.

The differential diagnosis of small cell carcinoma is vast, although many entities in the differential diagnosis are distinctly rare. The importance of accurate diagnosis is underscored by the therapeutic and prognostic implications heralded by the diagnosis of small cell carcinoma.

Some high-grade urothelial cancers have smaller cells and a diffuse growth pattern such that the possibility of small cell carcinoma is raised (efig 705). Alternatively, urothelial carcinomas may have a prominent lymphoid infiltrate mimicking "small cell" histology. Attention to the cytologic features and appropriate immunohistochemical support help one to arrive at the right diagnosis. Malignant lymphomas involving the bladder usually preserve the native architecture of the bladder but are widely invasive through the bladder wall. The nuclear features are usually distinct from small cell carcinoma, but a simple immunohistochemical panel (keratin, CD45, CD-20, CD-3, and chromogranin or synaptophysin) may be helpful. Distinction from small cell carcinoma is critical, because bladder lymphomas have a prolonged survival and different chemotherapy protocol than small cell carcinomas. Metastasis from a small cell carcinoma (e.g., from the lung) may be difficult to rule out on the basis of histology alone, although presence of a CIS component or concurrent usual bladder carcinoma (urothelial, squamous, or adenocarcinoma histology) is useful; metastatic small cell cancers from the lung to the bladder are rarely symptomatic. A more problematic situation is to rule out a direct extension of a small cell carcinoma from the prostate gland or uterus. Approximately half of prostate small cell carcinomas have at least a small component of conventional histology and, hence, prosate-specific antigen (PSA) or prostate-specific acid phosphatase (PSAP) staining in the better differentiated areas is helpful. In bladder small cell carcinomas, if there is an associated adenocarcinoma component it is usually of the enteric or signet ring cell type. If histology is not discriminatory, greater importance must be placed on clinical findings and imaging studies to determine the primary origin.

Large cell neuroendocrine carcinoma has a more discernible architecture such as organoid, nested, palisaded, or trabecular (52). Necrosis is common. The cells are larger, polygonal with low nuclear to cytoplasmic ratio and abundant eosinophilic cytoplasm. Mitotic activity is easily appreciable. Nucleoli are usually prominent, although they may be only focally present. The nuclear chromatin is usually more coarsely granular than small cell carcinoma. The very few reported cases have had a dismal outcome.

Tumors with the typical histology of carcinoid tumor are distinctly more rare than small cell carcinoma in the bladder (53,54). The organoid growth, distinct vasculature, uniform nuclear size, stippled chromatin, and abundant cytoplasm characteristic of the neoplasm are present in all cases, making this a readily recognizable tumor once it is considered.

UROTHELIAL CARCINOMA WITH UNUSUAL CYTOPLASMIC FEATURES

Plasmacytoid Urothelial Carcinoma

In the past few years, urothelial carcinomas with a striking resemblance to plasma cells have been described (Figs. 6.34, 6.35) (efigs 706–714). The tumor cells are arranged as single cells in a loose or myxoid stroma and have abundant eccentrically pronounced eosinophilic cytoplasm (55–57). Tumors are poorly differentiated, usually having a coexisting typical high-grade urothelial carcinoma or sarcomatoid carcinoma histology. Immunohistochemical reactions for cytokeratin are confirmatory for epithelial differentiation, ruling out a lymphoma or a melanoma, and may be required in limited or small specimens. There are too few cases to ascertain true prognostic significance, although most patients have a poor outcome because of the poor differentiation and the usually high grade and stage of cancer.

Urothelial Carcinoma with Rhabdoid Features

Only a few cases of extrarenal rhabdoid tumor involving the bladder have been reported (Fig. 6.36) (efigs 715–718). Patients have ranged in age from 2 to 84 years. Whereas in one case, rhabdoid differentiation was seen associated with

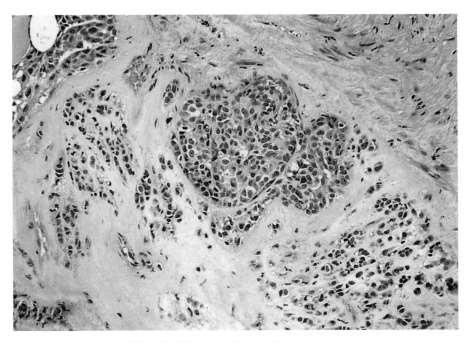

FIG. 6.34. Plasmacytoid urothelial carcinoma.

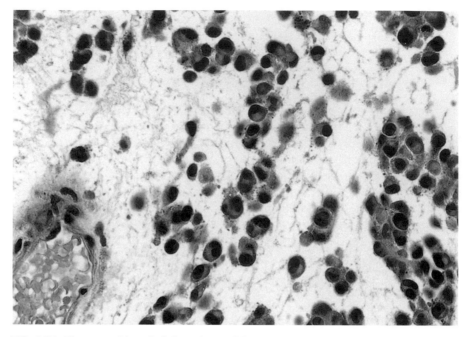

FIG. 6.35. Plasmacytoid urothelial carcinoma (higher magnification of Figure 6.34). Epithelial nature of tumor was highlighted by positive keratin stains (not shown).

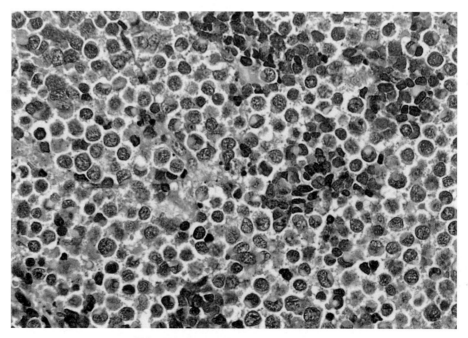

FIG. 6.36. Rhabdoid urothelial carcinoma.

a urothelial carcinoma, pure rhabdoid tumors of the bladder have also been reported, as have focal rhabdoid differentiation in a malignant fibrous histiocytoma (58–60).

Urothelial Carcinoma with Clear Cytoplasm

High-grade urothelial carcinomas may have abundant clear glycogenated cytoplasm (61,62) (Fig. 6.37) (efigs 719–722). This clear cell pattern is often focal but is rarely extensive such that the possibility of a metastatic renal cell carcinoma or extension from a prostatic adenocarcinoma with "hypernephroid" pattern may be considered. Clear cell adenocarcinoma of the bladder is also in the differential diagnosis, although it typically shows many patterns: for example, solid, cystic, glandular, or papillary. The presence of more typical areas of urothelial carcinoma is helpful to make the correct diagnosis, as is clinical history (62).

Lipid-Rich Urothelial Carcinoma

This cytoplasmic variation is extremely rare and is characterized by abundant lipid-distended cells mimicking signet ring cell adenocarcinoma (Fig. 6.38) (efig

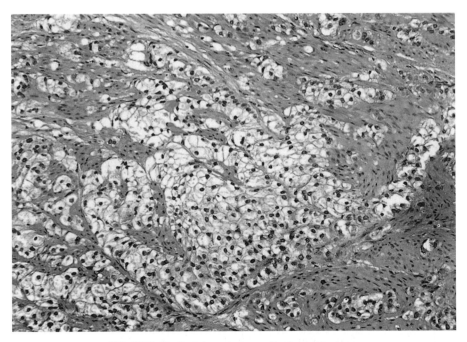

FIG. 6.37. Urothelial carcinoma with clear cytoplasm.

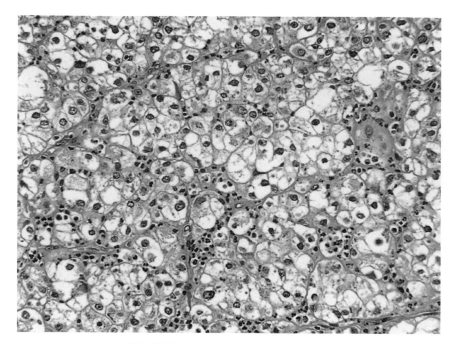

FIG. 6.38. Lipid-rich urothelial carcinoma.

723). In our experience, this pattern is focal or patchy, with other areas showing more typical areas of urothelial carcinoma.

UROTHELIAL CARCINOMA WITH TROPHOBLASTIC DIFFERENTIATION

This morphology in urothelial carcinoma is clearly rare and not more than 25 cases have been reported (1,63–65) (Figs. 6.39–6.41) (efigs 724–729). Although some of the early reports have described tumors that apparently were composed solely of tissue resembling choriocarcinoma, most of the cases reported in the past three decades have shown a mixture of urothelial carcinoma with trophoblastic elements (1). Thus, trophoblastic differentiation is recognized as a variant of urothelial carcinoma rather than a neoplasm of germ cell origin. Trophoblastic differentiation in urothelial carcinoma spans a spectrum from immunohistochemical expression for human chorionic gonadotropin (hCG) in an otherwise typical invasive high-grade urothelial carcinoma, to the presence of syncytiotrophoblasts, to the presence of focal areas resembling choriocarcinoma, and to the rare predominant or pure choriocarcinoma (63–67). Concurrent elevation of hCG in serum has been described. Immunohistochemistry often can detect hCG in typical urothelial carcinoma and some variants, including CIS. This is more common in high-grade carcinoma, approaching 33% of cases (Fig.

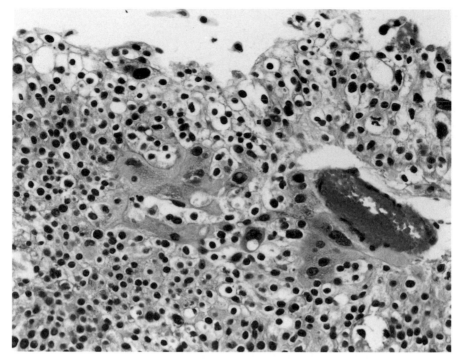

FIG. 6.39. Urothelial carcinoma with trophoblastic differentiation. Note scattered syncytiotrophoblasts.

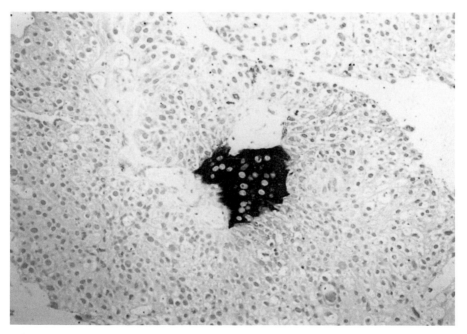

FIG. 6.40. Urothelial carcinoma with trophoblastic differentiation. Note scattered syncytiotrophoblasts as highlighted by stains for human chorionic gonadotropin.

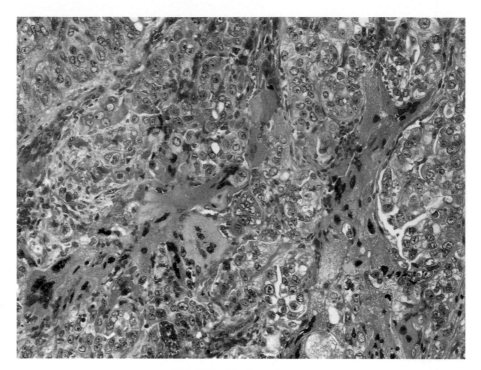

FIG. 6.41. Choriocarcinoma.

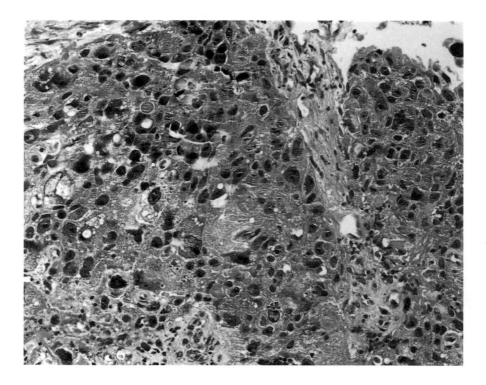

6.42) (efigs 730–732). Immunohistochemistry for hCG is not routinely performed, because the prognostic utility of this immunoreactivity is not established. The presence of syncytiotrophoblastic giant cells has been associated with a poor prognosis, with most reported patients dying within a year. For this reason, the presence of elements with trophoblastic morphology and some estimate as to their quantity may be reported.

UROTHELIAL CARCINOMA WITH UNUSUAL STROMAL REACTIONS

Pseudosarcomatous Stroma

Urothelial carcinomas may have a pseudosarcomatous stromal response in the primary or metastatic sites (38) (Fig. 6.43) (efigs 733, 734). In these cases, the stroma contains atypical mesenchymal cells that are similar to those seen in giant cell cystitis. The chief reason for their awareness is that they should not be misinterpreted as the biphasic component of sarcomatoid carcinoma. The superficially, very atypical appearing spindle cells often have abundant eosinophilic cytoplasm and pleomorphic hyperchromatic nuclei that have a degenerate appearance. The spindle cell component lacks mitotic activity or an expansile growth, and there is a lack of morphologic transition between the spindle cells and the carcinoma cells. This lesion is different from urothelial carcinoma with myxoid stroma, in which atypical cells are absent (efigs 735–737).

Osseous or Cartilaginous Metaplasia

The stroma of urothelial carcinomas or their metastases may rarely undergo osseous or cartilaginous metaplasia. This feature should not be mistaken for heterologous differentiation in a sarcomatoid carcinoma (2,37).

Osteoclast-Type Giant Cells

Giant cells resembling osteoclasts occasionally are present in the stroma of bladder carcinoma (Figs. 6.44, 6.45) (efigs 738–747). Rare cases of tumors with predominant osteoclast-type giant cell histology have been reported as osteoclastomas of the urinary bladder (68–72). Most experts believe that the giant cells are an unusual histiocytic component accompanying the carcinoma rather than being a separate neoplasm.

FIG. 6.42. Anaplastic urothelial carcinoma associated with markedly elevated serum human chorionic gonadotropin level. The tumor lacks cytotrophoblasts and syncytiotrophoblasts necessary for diagnosis of choriocarcinoma.

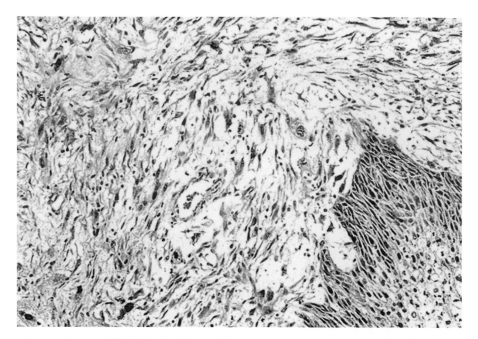

FIG. 6.43. Carcinoma with pseudosarcomatous stroma.

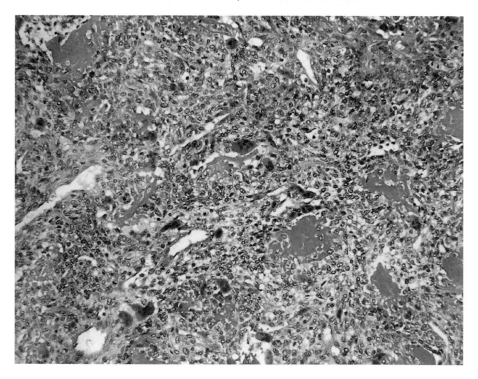

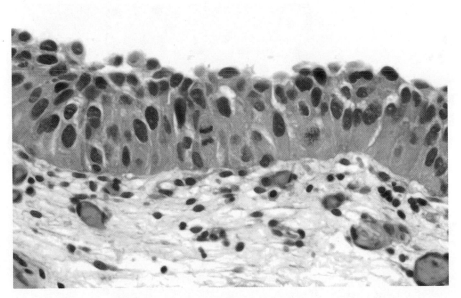

COLOR PLATE 1. Carcinoma in situ. (See efig 116.)

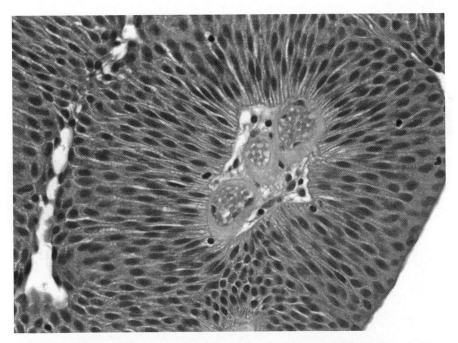

COLOR PLATE 2. Papillary urothelial neoplasm of low malignant potential. (See efig 283.)

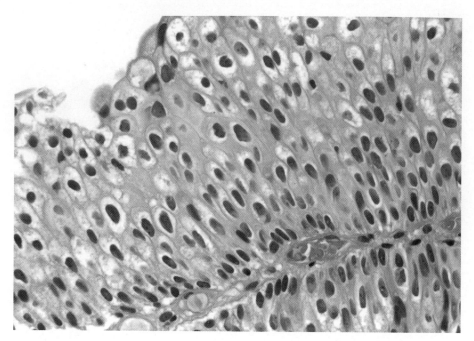

COLOR PLATE 3. Noninvasive low-grade papillary urothelial carcinoma. (See efig 319.)

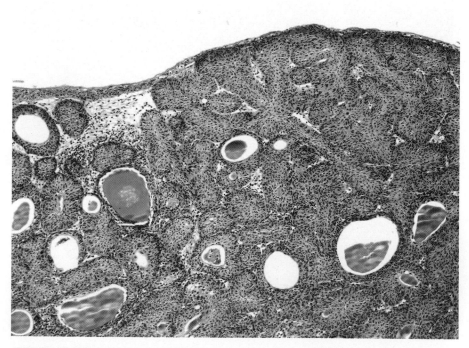

COLOR PLATE 4. Inverted urothelial papilloma with numerous colloid cysts. (See efig 453.)

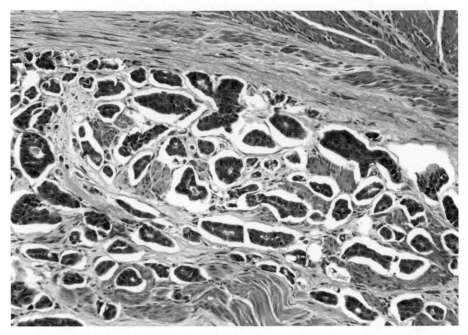

COLOR PLATE 5. Micropapillary carcinoma with muscularis propria invasion. (See efig 539.)

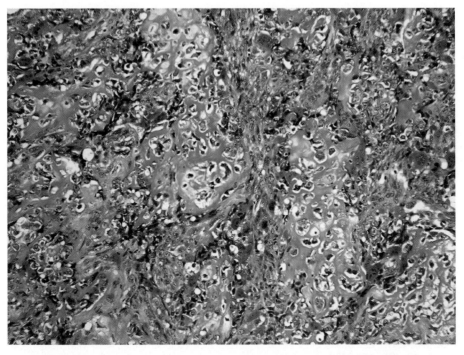

COLOR PLATE 6. Sarcomatoid carcinoma. Note malignant osteoid. (See efig 648.)

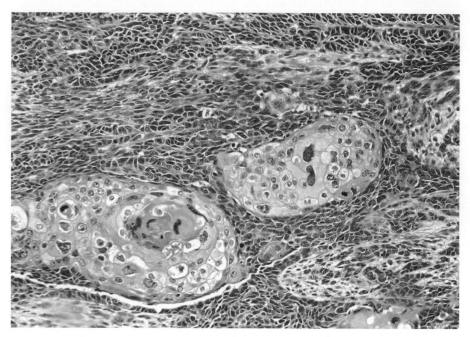

COLOR PLATE 7. Squamous cell carcinoma and small cell carcinoma. (See efig 665.)

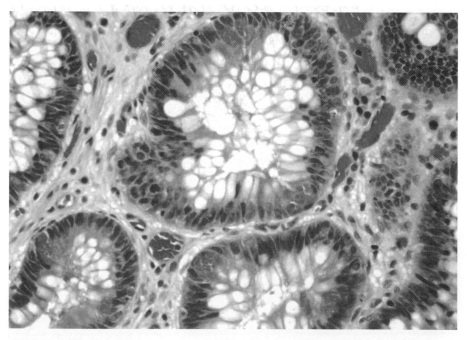

COLOR PLATE 8. Cystitis glandularis, intestinal type (colonic metaplasia) with Paneth cell metaplasia. (See efig 773.)

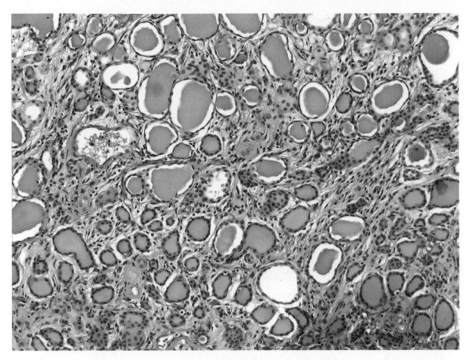

COLOR PLATE 9. Nephrogenic adenoma with thyroid-like secretions. (See efig 885.)

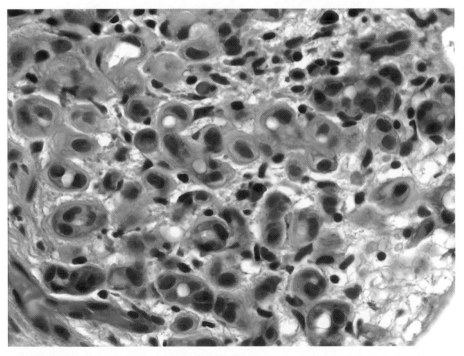

COLOR PLATE 10. Nephrogenic adenoma with signet ring cell–like features surrounded by hyaline membrane material. (See efig 890.)

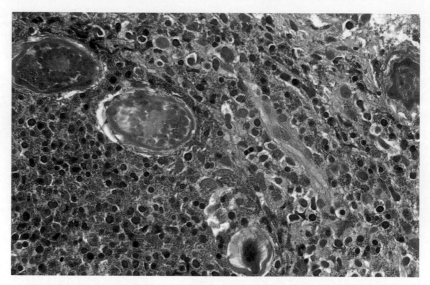

COLOR PLATE 11. Schistosomiasis with numerous eosinophils. (See efig 926.)

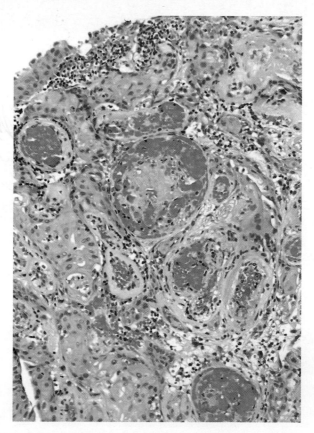

COLOR PLATE 12. Pseudocarcinomatous hyperplasia resulting from radiotherapy. Note urothelial nests surrounding fibrin and small vessels. (See efig 1019.)

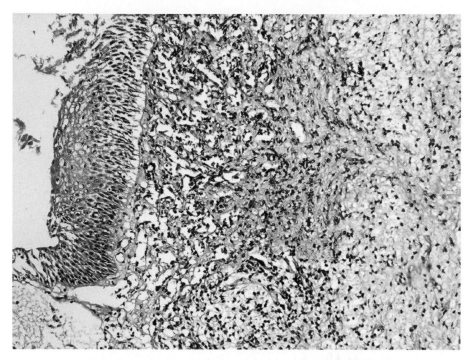

COLOR PLATE 13. Rhabdomyosarcoma with botryoid pattern.

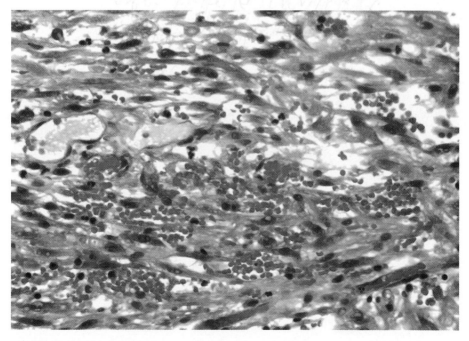

COLOR PLATE 14. Inflammatory myofibroblastic tumor with tissue culture fibroblast-like cells and extravasated red blood cells. (See efig 1091.)

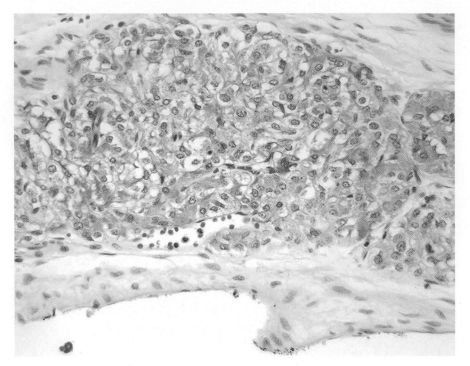

COLOR PLATE 15. Paraganglia. (See efig 1198.)

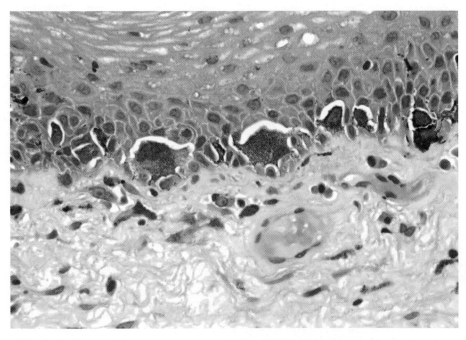

COLOR PLATE 16. Melanoma involving urothelial mucosa extending from vaginal primary. (See efig 1247.)

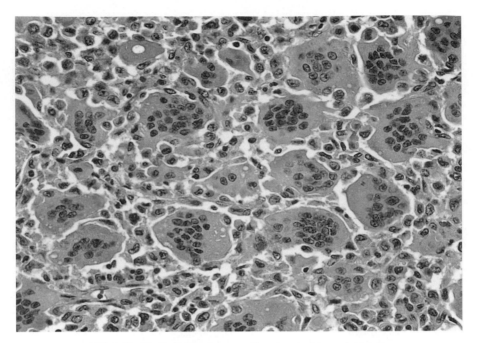

FIG. 6.45. Urothelial carcinoma with osteoclast-type giant cells.

GIANT CELL CARCINOMA/UNDIFFERENTIATED CARCINOMA

This is an undifferentiated carcinoma of the bladder that occasionally may be composed predominantly or purely of poorly differentiated, large, cohesive pleomorphic, multinucleated, and multinucleated anaplastic cells with abundant eosinophilic or amphophilic cytoplasm (1,2) (Fig. 6.46) (efigs 748–750). The tumor cells often contain multiple nucleoli and are similar to giant cell carcinomas seen in the lung and in other parts of the body. The high degree of nuclear anaplasia helps differentiate giant cell carcinoma from the osteoclast-type giant cells that may be seen in urothelial carcinoma. Other giant cells that may be seen with urothelial carcinoma include syncytiotrophoblastic giant cells or foreign body giant cells secondary to previous biopsy or resection.

Uncommonly, an epithelial tumor is found in the urinary bladder and consists of sheets of nondescript undifferentiated cells without squamous, urothelial, or glandular differentiation. Some authorities would classify these cases as large-cell undifferentiated carcinoma (Fig. 6.47) (efigs 705, 751–753). Others may

FIG. 6.44. Urothelial carcinoma with osteoclast-type giant cells.

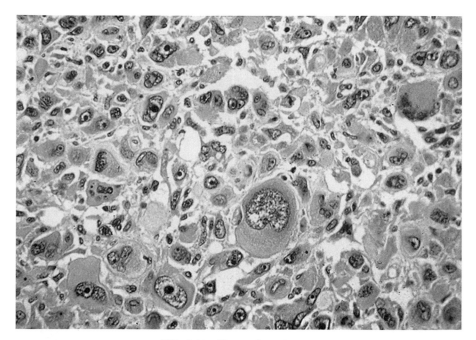

FIG. 6.46. Giant cell carcinoma.

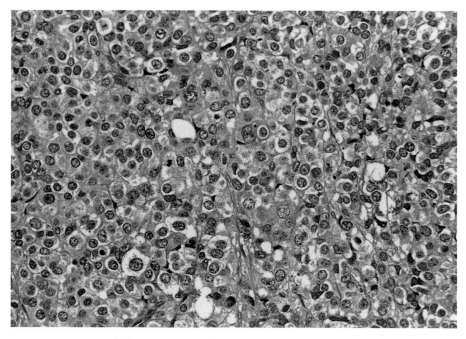

FIG. 6.47. Large cell undifferentiated carcinoma.

prefer to denote these lesions as high-grade urothelial carcinoma, given that this is the most common cancer within the bladder and that this pattern of tumor most likely represents the most poorly differentiated manifestation of usual urothclial carcinoma. There are currently no studies to determine whether there are any biologic differences in prognosis or treatment between high-grade urothelial carcinoma and "large cell undifferentiated" carcinoma. Until such data exist, either term used to describe such a lesion is appropriate.

SUMMARY

In summary, urothelial lesions have a pronounced ability for divergent differentiation. It is important that surgical pathologists be aware of this potential for multidirectional differentiation (so-called tumor plasticity), because it may have diagnostic, therapeutic, or prognostic implications (1,2).

Immunohistochemical methods are sometimes necessary to confirm whether a tumor, particularly one with variant histology, shows urothelial differentiation. Urothelial carcinomas are most frequently positive for high-molecular-weight cytokeratin (clone 34βE12), p63 (clone 4A4), and CK7. Urothelial carcinoma is often considered as a prototypic example of a CK7- and CK20-positive tumor, although only about half of invasive urothelial carcinomas are positive for CK20. Other novel markers include thrombomodulin (sensitive but not specific) and uroplakin III (specific but not sensitive) (22).

REFERENCES

1. Eble JN, Young RH. Carcinoma of the urinary bladder: a review of its diverse morphology. *Semin Diagn Pathol* 1997;14:98–108.
2. Amin MB, Murphy WM, Reuter VE, et al. Controversies in the pathology of transitional cell carcinoma of the urinary bladder. Part I, Chapter 1. In: Rosen PP, Fechner RE, eds. *Reviews of pathology*, vol 1. Chicago: ASCP Press, 1996:1–39.
3. Talbert WM, Young RH. Carcinomas of the urinary bladder with deceptively benign appearing foci—a report of three cases. *Am J Surg Pathol* 1989;13:374.
4. Murphy WM, Deana DG. The nested variant of transitional cell carcinoma: a clinicopathologic and immunohistochemical study of 44 cases. *Mod Pathol* 1992;5:240–243.
5. Young RH, Oliva E. Transitional carcinomas of the urinary bladder that may be underdiagnosed: a report of four cases exemplifying the homology between neoplastic and non-neoplastic transitional cell lesions. *Am J Surg Pathol* 1996;20:1148–1454.
6. Oliva E, Young RH. Nephrogenic adenoma of the urinary tract. A review of microscopic appearances of 80 cases with emphasis on unusual features. *Mod Pathol* 1995;8:722–730.
7. Cardillo M, Reuter VE, Lin O. Cytologic features of the nested variant of urothelial carcinoma: a study of seven cases. *Cancer* 2003;99:23–27.
8. Holmang S, Johansson SL. The nested variant of transitional cell carcinoma—a rare neoplasm with poor prognosis. *Scand J Urol Nephrol* 2001;35:102–105.
9. Drew PA, Furman J, Civantos F, et al. The nested variant of transitional cell carcinoma: an aggressive neoplasm with innocuous histology. *Mod Pathol* 1996;9:989–994.
10. Amin MB, Young RH. Intraepithelial lesions of the urinary bladder with a discussion of the histogenesis of urothelial neoplasia. *Semin Diagn Pathol* 1997;14:84–97.
11. Ro JY, Lapham R, Amin MB. Deceptively bland transitional cell carcinoma of the urinary bladder—further characterization of subtle and diagnostically treacherous patterns of invasion in urothelial neoplasia. *Adv Anat Pathol* 1997;4:244–251.

12. Young RH, Zukerberg LR. Microcystic transitional cell carcinomas of the urinary bladder: a report of four cases. *Am J Clin Pathol* 1991;96:635–639.
13. Paz A, Rath-Wolfson L, Lask D, et al. The clinical and histological features of transitional cell carcinoma of the bladder with microcysts: analysis of 12 cases. *Br J Urol* 1997;79:722–725.
14. Leroy X, Leteurtre E, De La Taille A, et al. Microcystic transitional cell carcinoma: a report of 2 cases arising in the renal pelvis. *Arch Pathol Lab Med* 2002;126:859–861.
15. Amin MB, Gomez JA, Young RH. Urothelial transitional cell carcinoma with endophytic growth patterns: a discussion of patterns of invasion and problems associated with assessment of invasion in 18 cases. *Am J Surg Pathol* 1997;21:1057–1068.
16. Terai A, Tamaki M, Hayashida H, et al. Bulky transitional cell carcinoma of bladder with inverted proliferation. *Int J Urol* 1996;3:316–319.
17. Amin MB, Ro JY, el-Sharkawy T, et al. Micropapillary variant of transitional cell carcinoma of the urinary bladder. Histologic pattern resembling ovarian papillary serous carcinoma. *Am J Surg Pathol* 1994;18:1224–1232.
18. Johansson SL, Borghede G, Holmang S. Micropapillary bladder carcinoma: a clinicopathological study of 20 cases. *J Urol* 1999;161:1798–1802.
19. Vera J, Marigil M, Garcia MD, et al. Micropapillary bladder carcinoma. *Virchows Arch* 2002;441:412–413.
20. Ylagan LR, Humphrey PA. Micropapillary variant of transitional cell carcinoma of the urinary bladder: a report of three cases with cytologic diagnosis in urine specimens. *Acta Cytol* 2001;45:599–604.
21. Maranchie JK, Bouyounes BT, Zhang PL, et al. Clinical and pathological characteristics of micropapillary transitional cell carcinoma: a highly aggressive variant. *J Urol* 2000;163:748–751.
22. Parker DC, Folpe AL, Bell J, et al. Potential utility of uroplakin III, thrombomodulin, high molecular weight cytokeratin, and cytokeratin 20 in noninvasive, invasive, and metastatic urothelial (transitional cell) carcinomas. *Am J Surg Pathol* 2003;27:1–10.
23. Amin MB, Ro JY, Lee KM, et al. Lymphoepithelioma-like carcinoma of urinary bladder. *Am J Surg Pathol* 1994;18:466–473.
24. Young RH, Eble JN. Lymphoepithelioma-like carcinoma of urinary bladder. *J Urol Pathol* 1993;1:63–67.
25. Ward JN, Dong WF, Pitts WR Jr. Lymphoepithelioma-like carcinoma of the bladder. *J Urol* 2002;167:2523–2524.
26. Lopez-Beltran A, Luque RJ, Vicioso L, et al. Lymphoepithelioma-like carcinoma of the urinary bladder: a clinicopathologic study of 13 cases. *Virchows Arch* 2001;438:552–557.
27. Holmang S, Borghede G, Johansson SL. Bladder carcinoma with lymphoepithelioma-like differentiation: a report of 9 cases. *J Urol* 1998;159:779–782.
28. Gulley ML, Amin MB, Nicholls JM, et al. Epstein-Barr virus is detected in undifferentiated nasopharyngeal carcinoma but not in lymphoepithelioma-like carcinoma of the urinary bladder. *Hum Pathol* 1995;26:1207–1214.
29. Zuckerberg LR, Harris NL, Young RH. Carcinomas of the urinary bladders simulating malignant lymphoma. *Am J Surg Pathol* 1991;15:569–576.
30. Ro JY, Ayala AG, Wishnow K, et al. Sarcomatoid bladder carcinoma: clinicopathological and immunohistochemical study of 44 cases. *Surg Pathol* 1988;1:359.
31. Young RH, Wick MR, Mills SE. Sarcomatoid carcinoma of the urinary bladder: a clinicopathological analysis of 12 cases and review of literature. *Am J Clin Pathol* 1988;90:653–661.
32. Ikegami H, Iwasaki H, Ohjimi Y, et al. Sarcomatoid carcinoma of the urinary bladder: a clinicopathologic and immunohistochemical analysis of 14 patients. *Hum Pathol* 2000;31:332–340.
33. Lopez-Beltran A, Pacelli A, Rothenberg HJ, et al. Carcinosarcoma and sarcomatoid carcinoma of the bladder: clinicopathological study of 41 cases. *J Urol* 1998;159:1497–1503.
34. Jones EC, Young RH. Myxoid and sclerosing sarcomatoid transitional cell carcinoma of the urinary bladder: a clinicopathologic and immunohistochemical study of 25 cases. *Mod Pathol* 1997;10:908–916.
35. Torenbeek R, Blomjous CE, de Bruin PC, et al. Sarcomatoid carcinoma of the urinary bladder. Clinicopathologic analysis of 18 cases with immunohistochemical and electron microscopic findings. *Am J Surg Pathol* 1994;18:241–249.
36. Ro JY, el-Naggar AK, Amin MB, et al. Pseudosarcomatous fibromyxoid tumor of the urinary bladder and prostate: immunohistochemical, ultrastructural, and DNA flow cytometric analyses of nine cases. *Hum Pathol* 1993;24:1203–1210.

37. Gazaigne J, Mozziconacci JG, Provendier B, et al. Sarcomatoid carcinoma of the bladder with major osseous metaplasia. *Prog Urol* 1998;8:1051–1053.
38. Young RH, Wick MR. Transitional cell carcinoma of the urinary bladder with pseudosarcomatous stroma. *Am J Clin Pathol* 1988;90:216–219.
39. Angulo JC, Lopez JI, Sanchez-Chapado M, et al. Small cell carcinoma of the urinary bladder. *J Urol Pathol* 1996;5:1–19.
40. Mills SE, Wolfe JT 3rd, Weiss MA, et al. Small cell undifferentiated carcinoma of the urinary bladder. A light-microscopic, immunocytochemical, and ultrastructural study of 12 cases. *Am J Surg Pathol* 1987;11:606–617.
41. Weiss MA. Small cell carcinomas of the urinary tract. *Arch Pathol Lab Med* 1993;117:237–238.
42. Trias I, Algaba F, Condom E, et al. Small cell carcinoma of the urinary bladder. Presentation of 23 cases and review of 134 published cases. *Eur Urol* 2001;39:85–90.
43. Holmang S, Borghede G, Johansson SL. Primary small cell carcinoma of the bladder: a report of 25 cases. *J Urol* 1995;153:1820–1822.
44. Lopez JI, Angulo JC, Flores N, et al. Small cell carcinoma of the urinary bladder. A clinicopathological study of six cases. *Br J Urol* 1994;73:43–49.
45. Grignon DJ, Ro JY, Ayala AG, et al. Small cell carcinoma of the urinary bladder. A clinicopathologic analysis of 22 cases. *Cancer* 1992;69:527–536.
46. Blomjous CE, Vos W, De Voogt HJ, et al. Small cell carcinoma of the urinary bladder. A clinicopathologic, morphometric, immunohistochemical, and ultrastructural study of 18 cases. *Cancer* 1989;64:1347–1357.
47. Eusebi V, Damiani S, Pasquinelli G, et al. Small cell neuroendocrine carcinoma with skeletal muscle differentiation: report of three cases. *Am J Surg Pathol* 2000;24:223–230.
48. Fujita K, Nishimura K, Nonomura N, et al. Early stage small cell carcinoma of the urinary bladder. *Int J Urol* 2001;8:643–644.
49. Lohrisch C, Murray N, Pickles T, et al. Small cell carcinoma of the bladder: long term outcome with integrated chemoradiation. *Cancer* 1999;86:2346–2352.
50. Bastus R, Caballero JM, Gonzalez G, et al. Small cell carcinoma of the urinary bladder treated with chemotherapy and radiotherapy: results in five cases. *Eur Urol* 1999;35:323–326.
51. Agoff SN, Lamps LW, Philip AT, et al. Thyroid transcription factor-1 is expressed in extrapulmonary small cell carcinomas but not in other extrapulmonary neuroendocrine tumors. *Mod Pathol* 2000;13:238–242.
52. Hailemariam S, Gaspert A, Komminoth P, et al. Primary, pure, large-cell neuroendocrine carcinoma of the urinary bladder. *Mod Pathol* 1998;11:1016–1020.
53. Martignoni G, Eble JN. Carcinoid tumors of the urinary bladder. Immunohistochemical study of 2 cases and review of the literature. *Arch Pathol Lab Med* 2003;127:e22–24.
54. Akimov OV, Chukin SE. Malignant carcinoid of the urinary bladder. *Arkh Patol* 2002; 64:41–42.
55. Tamboli P, Amin MB, Mohsin SK, et al. Plasmacytoid variant of non-papillary urothelial carcinoma (UC). *Mod Pathol* 2000;13:107A.
56. Zhang XM, Elhosseiny A, Melamed MR. Plasmacytoid urothelial carcinoma of the bladder. A case report and the first description of urinary cytology. *Acta Cytol* 2002;46:412–416.
57. Sahin AA, Myhre M, Ro JY, et al. Plasmacytoid transitional cell carcinoma. Report of a case with initial presentation mimicking multiple myeloma. *Acta Cytol* 1991;35:277–280.
58. Inagaki T, Nagata M, Kaneko M, et al. Carcinosarcoma with rhabdoid features of the urinary bladder in a 2-year-old girl: possible histogenesis of stem cell origin. *Pathol Int* 2000;50:973–978.
59. Harris M, Eyden BP, Joglekar VM. Rhabdoid tumour of the bladder: a histological, ultrastructural and immunohistochemical study. *Histopathology* 1987;11:1083–1092.
60. Egawa S, Uchida T, Koshiba K, et al. Malignant fibrous histiocytoma of the bladder with focal rhabdoid tumor differentiation. *J Urol* 1994;151:154–156.
61. Kotliar SN, Wood CA, Schaeffer AJ, et al. Transitional cell carcinoma exhibiting clear cell features: a differential diagnosis for clear cell adenocarcinoma of the urinary tract. *Arch Pathol Lab Med* 1995;119:79–81.
62. Oliva E, Amin MB, Jimenez R, et al. Clear cell carcinoma of the urinary bladder: a report and comparison of four tumors of mullerian origin and nine of probable urothelial origin with discussion of histogenesis and diagnostic problems. *Am J Surg Pathol* 2002;26:190–197.
63. Tinkler SD, Roberts JT, Robinson MC, et al. Primary choriocarcinoma of the urinary bladder: a case report. *Clin Oncol (R Coll Radiol)* 1996;8:59–61.

64. Yokoyama S, Hayashida Y, Nagahama J, et al. Primary and metaplastic choriocarcinoma of the bladder. A report of two cases. *Acta Cytol* 1992;36:176–182.
65. Sievert K, Weber EA, Herwig R, et al. Pure primary choriocarcinoma of the urinary bladder with long-term survival. *Urology* 2000;56:856.
66. Dirnhofer S, Koessler P, Ensinger C, et al. Production of trophoblastic hormones by transitional cell carcinoma of the bladder: association to tumor stage and grade. *Hum Pathol* 1998;29:377–382.
67. Ozkardes H, Ergen A, Ozen HA, et al. Immunohistochemical detection of beta-human chorionic gonadotropin in urothelial carcinoma. *Int Urol Nephrol* 1991;23:5–11.
68. Amir G, Rosenmann E. Osteoclast-like giant cell tumour of the urinary bladder. *Histopathology* 1990;17:413-418.
69. Lidgi S, Embon OM, Turani H, et al. Giant cell reparative granuloma of the bladder associated with transitional cell carcinoma. *J Urol* 1989;142:120–122.
70. Kitazawa M, Kobayashi H, Ohnishi Y, et al. Giant cell tumor of the bladder associated with transitional cell carcinoma. *J Urol* 1985;133:472–475.
71. Zukerberg LR, Armin AR, Pisharodi L, et al. Transitional cell carcinoma of the urinary bladder with osteoclast-type giant cells: a report of two cases and review of the literature. *Histopathology* 1990; 17:407–411.
72. O'Connor RC, Hollowell CM, Laven BA, et al. Recurrent giant cell carcinoma of the bladder. *J Urol* 2002;167:1784.

7

Conventional Morphologic, Prognostic, and Predictive Factors and Reporting of Bladder Cancer

The traditional morphologic, prognostic, and predictive factors for bladder cancer vary according to the type of bladder cancer presentation in the patient: noninvasive papillary tumors, primary urothelial carcinoma in situ (CIS), or invasive urothelial carcinoma (1). The prognostic factors are, hence, discussed separately for each category and are summarized in Table 7.1. There are several molecular and chromosomal markers (e.g., loss of chromosome 9, loss of material on chromosome 17, p53, retinoblastoma tumor suppressor gene status) that are likely to complement traditional morphologic markers in the future, but these are not routinely used in current surgical pathology practice (2). Additionally, clinical parameters (e.g., comorbid disease) as well as clinical presentation (e.g., increased frequency of recurrence and short interval between recurrences) influence progression to grade and stage.

TABLE 7.1. *Morphologic prognostic and predictive factors of bladder cancer*

Noninvasive papillary tumors
    Histologic grade
    Size of tumor
    Multifocality
    Status of nonpapillary urothelium—carcinoma in situ (CIS)
Urothelial CIS
    Mode of presentation—primary (*de novo*) or secondary
    Multifocality
    Failure to respond to typical therapy
Invasive urothelial carcinoma
    Depth of invasion in bladder wall (pT stage)
    Lymph node involvement (pN stage)
    Involvement of prostate gland and seminal vesicles
    Histologic type
    Histologic grade (controversial)
    Vascular–lymphatic invasion (controversial)
    Surgical margin status for invasive carcinoma
    Multifocality and CIS of urethra or ureters

NONINVASIVE PAPILLARY TUMORS

Histologic Grade

Histologic grade is a powerful prognostic factor for recurrence and progression in noninvasive tumors. Urothelial papilloma has the lowest risk for either recurrence or progression, whereas papillary urothelial neoplasm of low malignant potential has a risk for recurrence but still has a low risk for progression. Patients with papilloma and neoplasms of low malignant potential have essentially a normal age-related life expectancy (see Chapter 3). Progression risk in grade and stage and mortality increases from low-grade carcinomas to high-grade carcinomas (3,4).

Size of Tumor

Large tumors (often greater than 3 cm) are at an increased risk for recurrence and progression (5,6).

Multifocality

Patients with multifocal tumors in the bladder and involving other regions of the urothelial tract (ureters and urethra) are at increased risk for recurrence, progression, or death due to disease (5,7,8).

Urothelial Carcinoma In Situ in Nonpapillary Mucosa

Although the impact of the presence of dysplasia in the nonpapillary urothelium is controversial as a prognostic factor and at best may represent a marker of urothelial instability, the presence of urothelial CIS is a known adverse prognostic factor in terms of recurrence and progression (9,10).

UROTHELIAL CARCINOMA IN SITU

Patients with primary (de novo) CIS are more likely to have no evidence of disease (62% versus 45%) and are less likely to progress (28% versus 59%) or die of disease (7% versus 45%) (11). Patients with multifocal disease and those who fail to respond to intravesical therapy have a worse outcome (1,11,12).

INVASIVE UROTHELIAL CARCINOMA

Depth of Invasion in Bladder Wall

Once a urothelial carcinoma is invasive, the most seminal prognostic factor is the American Joint Committee on Cancer/International Union against Cancer pathologic stage (13) (Table 7.2). The pT system of staging has excellent correlation with prognosis and distinguishes distinct prognostic groups. Tumors invasive into the lamina propria (pT1) have a better survival than tumors invasive into the muscularis propria (pT2), with poor survival for tumors with extraves-

TABLE 7.2. *American Joint Committee on Cancer staging system for bladder cancer*

Primary tumor (T)[a]

TX	Primary tumor cannot be assessed
T0	No evidence of primary tumor
Ta	Noninvasive papillary carcinoma
Tis	Carcinoma in situ: "flat tumor"
T1	Tumor invades subepithelial connective tissue
T2	Tumor invades muscle
T2a	Tumor invades superficial muscle (inner half)
T2b	Tumor invades deep muscle (outer half)
T3	Tumor invades perivesical tissue
T3a	Microscopically
T3b	Macroscopically (extravesicular mass)
T4	Tumor invades any of the following: prostate, uterus, vagina, pelvic wall, or abdominal wall
T4a	Tumor invades prostate, uterus, or vagina
T4b	Tumor invades pelvic wall or abdominal wall

Regional lymph nodes (N)
Regional lymph nodes are those within the true pelvis; all others are distant nodes.

NX	Regional lymph nodes cannot be assessed
N0	No regional lymph node metastasis
N1	Metastasis in a single lymph node, 2 cm or less in greatest dimension
N2	Metastasis in a single lymph node, more than 2 cm but not more than 5 cm in greatest dimension, or multiple lymph nodes, none more than 5 cm in greatest dimension
N3	Metastasis in a lymph node more than 5 cm in greatest dimension

Distant metastasis (M)

MX	Distant metastasis cannot be assessed
M0	No distant metastasis
M1	Distant metastasis

TNM stage grouping: bladder

Stage 0a	Ta	N0	M0
Stage 0is	Tis	N0	M0
Stage I	T1	N0	M0
Stage II	T2a	N0	M0
	T2b	N0	M0
Stage III	T3a	N0	M0
	T3b	N0	M0
Stage IV	T4a	N0	M0
	T4b	N0	M0
	Any T	N1,2,3	M0
	Any T	Any N	M1

[a]The suffix "m" should be added to the appropriate T category to indicate multiple tumors. The suffix "is" may be added to any T to indicate the presence of associated carcinoma in situ.
Adapted from Greene FL, Page DL, Fleming ID, et al. *AJCC cancer staging manual.* 6th ed. New York: Springer, 2002:369.

icular extension (pT3, pT4) (1,14–16). Although substaging of urothelial tumors (pT1a—tumors invasive up to muscularis mucosae; pT1b—tumors invasive into or beyond muscularis mucosae) has shown prognostic value, it is currently not recommended because it may not always be possible to substage pT1 tumors due to absence of muscularis mucosae in some bladders or because of a lack of orientation in transurethral resection specimens precluding orientation (2).

Lymph Node Involvement

Patients with regional spread of tumor (node-positive) have a poor prognosis. The 5-year recurrence-free survival of patients is 35%, and the 5-year overall survival is 31% (16). Immunohistochemical detection of micrometastasis has no established prognostic value (17).

Involvement of Prostate Gland and Seminal Vesicles

The prostate ducts and acini and seminal vesicular epithelium may be involved by urothelial carcinoma extending along the luminal aspect (mucosal spread of CIS) (18–20). CIS of prostate ducts and acini predicts a high recurrence on a stage-adjusted basis but is not equivalent to pT4 disease. Invasion of the prostatic or seminal vesicle stroma secondary to CIS is usually a microscopic disease but when present portends a very poor prognosis. The precise stage designation for this form of invasion is not recognized in the current TNM (tumor, node, metastasis) classification. Involvement of prostatic stroma may also be due to direct extension from a transmurally invasive bladder cancer (pT4), which is also associated with dismal prognosis (18,19).

Histologic Type

Aberrant differentiation (squamous or glandular) in urothelial carcinoma has no known prognostic significance except that the frequency and extent is directly proportional to the grade of urothelial carcinoma (1,20–22). Pure squamous carcinomas and adenocarcinomas tend to present at higher stage but, when corrected for stage, have an outcome similar to urothelial carcinoma of similar stage. Nested variant of urothelial carcinoma, micropapillary urothelial carcinoma, sarcomatoid carcinoma (carcinosarcoma), and small cell carcinoma are histologic patterns associated with poor outcome (see Chapter 6). The diagnoses of urachal adenocarcinoma, lymphoepithelioma-like carcinoma, and small cell carcinoma have additional therapeutic relevance (see Chapters 6 and 8) for example, urachal carcinomas are often treated with partial cystectomy, excision of urachal tract, and umbilectomy, in contrast to primary mucosal bladder muscle invasive adenocarcinomas, which are usually treated with radical cystectomy (23).

Histologic Grade

Once the tumor is invasive, the importance of histologic grade is controversial and not shown to be of great value. There is, in fact, often an outcome paradox; for example, nested variants, which may be low grade, have a poor outcome (24).

Vascular–Lymphatic Invasion

The importance of this feature is controversial because retraction artifact around a tumor is often overdiagnosed as such. Unequivocal invasion into endothelium-lined spaces has been shown to be significant in univariate analysis (25,26).

Surgical Margin Status

Presence of invasive carcinoma at the resection margin is an adverse prognostic parameter, primarily for local recurrence.

Multifocality and Carcinoma In Situ of Urethra or Ureters

Patients with multifocal high-grade papillary or invasive tumors or multifocal CIS are at an increased risk for recurrence. Presence of CIS at the urethral margin at cystoprostatectomy may be an indication for urethrectomy.

REPORTING OF BLADDER CANCER

The elements that should be included in the surgical pathology report must have prognostic significance and should likely be important for patient management. Checklists for reporting bladder cancer have been developed by the College of American Pathologists and the Association of Directors of Anatomic and Surgical Pathology (27,28). Table 7.3 summarizes the essential elements to be

TABLE 7.3. *Elements to be included in bladder cancer surgical pathology reports*

Biopsy/transurethral resection
Essential
Histologic type (e.g., urothelial, squamous cell)
Histologic grade [WHO(2003)/ISUP for urothelial carcinoma]
Pathologic stage (pT) (only pTa, PT1, or pT2)
Presence or absence of muscularis propria
Presence or absence of urothelial carcinoma in situ (CIS)
Optional
Configuration of tumor: e.g., papillary, ulcerative, solid
Unequivocal vascular–lymphatic invasion
Urothelial dysplasia
Other benign or proliferative, inflammatory, or therapy-related changes
Cystoprostatectomy/anterior exenteration
Essential
Histologic type (e.g., urothelial, squamous cell)
Histologic grade [WHO(2003)/ISUP for urothelial carcinoma]
Pathologic stage (pT and pN status)
Presence or absence of urothelial CIS
Involvement of prostate
Direct extension
Involvement of prostatic ducts and acini without stromal invasion
Involvement of prostatic ducts and acini with stromal invasion
Direct involvement of adjacent viscera (exenteration specimen)
Margins of excision for CIS (mention all negative and positive margins)
Margins of excision for invasive carcinoma (mention all negative and positive margins)
Optional
Configuration of tumor: e.g., papillary, flat, ulcerative, solid
Unequivocal vascular–lymphatic invasion
Multifocal tumors
Urothelial dysplasia
Other benign or proliferative, inflammatory, or therapy-related changes

ISUP, International Society of Urological Pathology; WHO, World Health Organization.

reported in biopsy and transurethral resection and in radical cystectomy and cystoprostatectomy specimens.

REFERENCES

1. Reuter VE. Bladder. Risk and prognostic factors—a pathologist's perspective. *Urol Clin North Am* 1999;26:481–492.
2. Jimenez RE, Keane TE, Hardy HT, et al. pT1 urothelial carcinoma of the bladder: criteria for diagnosis, pitfalls, and clinical implications. *Adv Anat Pathol* 2000;7:13–25.
3. Desai S, Lim SD, Jimenez RE, et al. Relationship of cytokeratin 20 and CD44 protein expression with WHO/ISUP grade in pTa and pT1 papillary urothelial neoplasia. *Mod Pathol* 2000;13:1315–1323.
4. Samaratunga H, Makarov DV, Epstein JI. Comparison of WHO/ISUP and WHO classification of non-invasive papillary urothelial neoplasms for risk of progression. *Urology* 2002;60:315–319.
5. Millan-Rodriguez F, Chechile-Toniolo G, Salvador-Bayarri J, et al. Multivariate analysis of the prognostic factors of primary superficial bladder cancer. *J Urol* 2000;163:73–78.
6. Heney NM, Ahmed S, Flanagan MJ, et al. Superficial bladder cancer: progression and recurrence. *J Urol* 1983;130:1083–1086.
7. Lutzeyer W, Rubben H, Dahm H. Prognostic parameters in superficial bladder cancer: an analysis of 315 cases. *J Urol* 1982;127:250–252.
8. Millan-Rodriguez F, Chechile-Toniolo G, Salvador-Bayarri J, et al. Upper urinary tract tumors after primary superficial bladder tumors: prognostic factors and risk groups. *J Urol* 2000;164:1183–1187.
9. Bono AV, Benvenuti C, Damiano G, et al. Results of transurethral resection and intravesical doxoru-bicin prophylaxis in patients with TIG3 bladder cancer. *Urology* 1994;44:329–334.
10. Nixon RG, Chang SS, Lafleur BJ, et al. Carcinoma in situ and tumor multifocality predict the rise of prostatic urethral involvement at radical cystectomy in men with transitional cell carcinoma of the bladder. *J Urol* 2002;167:502–505.
11. Orozco RE, Martin AA, Murphy WM. Carcinoma in situ of the urinary bladder. Clues to host involvement in human carcinogenesis. *Cancer* 1994;74:115–122.
12. Amin MB, McKenney JK. An approach to the diagnosis of flat intraepithelial lesions of the urinary bladder using the World Health Organization/ International Society of Urological Pathology consensus classification system. *Adv Anat Pathol* 2002;9:222–232.
13. Sobin LH, Wittekind C. *UICC TNM Classification of malignant tumours*, 6th ed. New York: Wiley-Liss, 2002.
14. Pagano F, Bassi P, Galetti TP. Results of contemporary radical cystectomy for invasive bladder cancer. A clinicopathological study with an emphasis on the inadequacy of the tumor, nodes, and metastases classification. *J Urol* 1991;145:45–50.
15. Richie JP, Skinner DG, Kaufman JJ. Radical cystectomy for carcinoma of the bladder: 16 years experience. *J Urol* 1975;113:186–189.
16. Stein JP, Lieskovsky G, Cote R, et al. Radical cystectomy in the treatment of invasive bladder cancer: long-term results in 1,054 patients. *J Clin Oncol* 2001;19:666–675.
17. Yang XJ, Lecksell K, Epstein JI. Can immunohistochemistry enhance the detection of micrometastases in pelvic lymph nodes from patients with high-grade urothelial carcinoma of the bladder? *Am J Clin Pathol* 1999;112:649–653.
18. Esrig D, Freeman JA, Elmajian DA, et al. Transitional cell carcinoma involving the prostate with a proposed staging classification for stromal invasion. *J Urol* 1996;156:1071–1076.
19. Ro JY, Ayala AG, el-Naggar A, et al. Seminal vesicle involvement by in situ and invasive transitional cell carcinoma of the bladder. *Am J Surg Pathol* 1987;11:951–958.
20. Amin MB, Murphy WM, Reuter VE, et al. A symposium on controversies in the pathology of transitional cell carcinomas of the urinary bladder, Part II. *Anat Pathol* 1997;2:71–110.
21. Eble JN, Young RH. Carcinoma of the urinary bladder: a review of its diverse morphology. *Semin Diagn Pathol* 1997;14:98–108.
22. Amin MB, Murphy WM, Reuter VE, et al. A symposium on controversies in the pathology of transitional cell carcinomas of the urinary bladder. Part I. *Anat Pathol* 1996;1:1–39.
23. Grignon DJ, Ro JY, Ayala AG, et al. Primary adenocarcinoma of the urinary bladder. A clinicopathologic analysis of 72 cases. *Cancer* 1991;67:2165–2172.
24. Jimenez RE, Gheiler E, Oskanian P, et al. Grading the invasive component of urothelial carcinoma of the bladder and its relationship with progression-free survival. *Am J Surg Pathol* 2000;24:980–987.

25. Heney NM, Proppe K, Prout GR Jr, et al. Invasive bladder cancer: tumor configuration, lymphatic invasion and survival. *J Urol* 1983;130:895–897.
26. Shipley WU, Rose MA, Perrone TL, et al. Full-dose irradiation for patients with invasive bladder carcinoma: clinical and histological factors prognostic of improved survival. *J Urol* 1985;134:679–683.
27. Murphy WM, Crissman JD, Johansson SL, et al. Association of Directors of Anatomic and Surgical Pathology. Recommendations for the reporting of urinary bladder specimens containing bladder neoplasms. *Am J Clin Pathol* 1996;106:568–570.
28. Amin MB, Srigley JR, Grignon DJ, et al. Protocol for the examination of specimens from patients with carcinoma of the urinary bladder, ureter, and renal pelvis. *Arch Pathol Lab Med* (*in press*).

8

Glandular Lesions

CYSTITIS GLANDULARIS (INTESTINAL TYPE)

In some cases, the epithelial lining of von Brunn nests and cystitis cystica undergo glandular metaplasia, giving rise to what is called *cystitis glandularis* (1,2). The cells become cuboidal or columnar and mucin secreting, taking on the appearance of intestinal-type goblet cells. This variant is called *cystitis glandularis with intestinal metaplasia* (colonic metaplasia) (Figs. 8.1–8.4) (Color Plate 8) (efigs 754–778). The change may be focal or may diffusely replace the lining

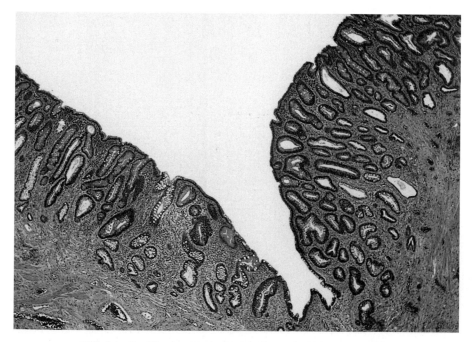

FIG. 8.1. Cystitis glandularis, intestinal type (colonic metaplasia).

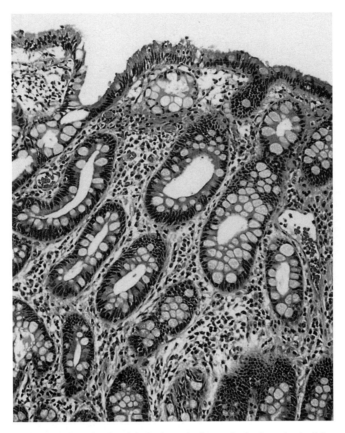

FIG. 8.2. Cystitis glandularis, intestinal type (colonic metaplasia).

urothelium, both presenting as flat or minimally distorted mucosa. Some cases of intestinal metaplasia may be associated with abundant mucin extravasation and may present as symptomatic mass lesions. Although there is overlap between some examples of colonic metaplasia and well-differentiated adenocarcinoma in some of the histologic features (dissecting mucin, infiltration of muscularis propria, atypia, and mitoses), the degree and extent of these findings differ between the two conditions (3,4). In contrast to the extensive mucinous pools seen in some adenocarcinomas, florid colonic metaplasia has only focal areas of mucin extravasation and typically is devoid of neoplastic cells within mucin pools (Fig. 8.5). Whereas adenocarcinomas typically show deep muscle invasion, the muscle invasion seen in colonic metaplasia tends to be more limited. Although rare adenocarcinomas may show bland cytology, most have areas of the tumor with overt cytologic atypia. The atypia seen in colonic metaplasia is negligible and mitoses, although frequent in adenocarcinoma, are found only

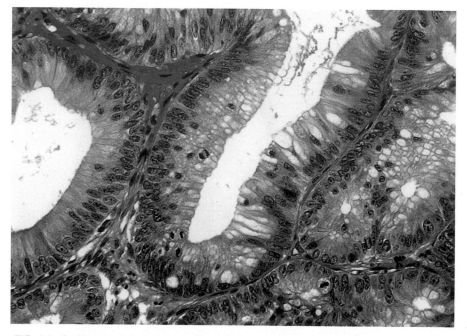

FIG. 8.3. Cystitis glandularis, intestinal type (colonic metaplasia) with adenomatous change.

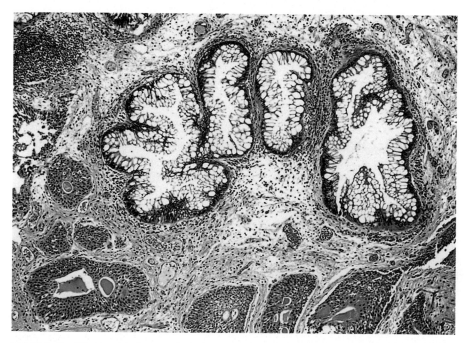

FIG. 8.4. Cystitis glandularis, intestinal type (colonic metaplasia). Note nonintestinal type cystitis cystica et glandularis (bottom).

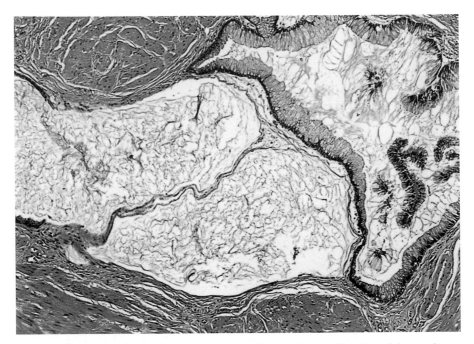

FIG. 8.5. Cystitis glandularis, intestinal type (colonic metaplasia) with extracellular mucinous pools dissecting muscularis propria.

rarely in colonic metaplasia. Other cases of adenocarcinoma that are less differentiated show signet cells and necrosis, which are not found in colonic metaplasia. Long-term follow-up of cases of colonic metaplasia has confirmed a benign behavior (5).

Glandular metaplasia may also occur within surface urothelium, usually as a response to chronic inflammation or irritation, such as in cases of uncorrected bladder extrophy (6,7). The epithelium is composed of tall columnar cells with mucin-secreting goblet cells, strikingly similar to colonic or small intestinal epithelium in which one might identify even Paneth cells.

VILLOUS ADENOMA

Glandular lesions occurring in the bladder and urethra are analogous to glandular lesions seen in the intestinal tract, both in terms of types of lesion and in their morphology. The full spectrum of lesions seen in the bladder and urethra include villous adenoma, villous adenoma with in situ adenocarcinoma, villous adenoma with infiltrating adenocarcinoma, and infiltrating adenocarcinoma without villous adenoma. Villous adenomas and adenocarcinomas in the bladder occur in one of two general locations. They may arise within the urachus such

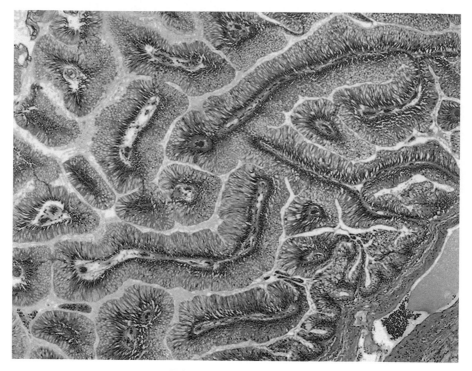

FIG. 8.6. Villous adenoma.

that they are seen at the dome or anterior wall of the bladder where they may present as a painful suprapubic mass. Or, glandular lesions arise in the bladder from a process of metaplasia in which they may occur anywhere in the bladder, typically near the trigone.

For both villous adenoma and adenocarcinoma of the bladder, there is a male predominance. Patients with villous adenoma or adenocarcinoma may present with nonspecific findings or, occasionally, with mucosuria. If the lesion is pure villous adenoma with or without in situ adenocarcinoma and the lesion is entirely resected, then the prognosis is excellent (8–12) (Figs. 8.6–8.8) (efigs 779–798). However, if the lesion has been only subtotally removed, especially in the setting of coexistent in situ adenocarcinoma, the tumors have the potential to progress to infiltrating adenocarcinoma. Because infiltrating adenocarcinoma is

FIG. 8.8. Villous adenoma of urachus with focal ruptured mucinous pools.

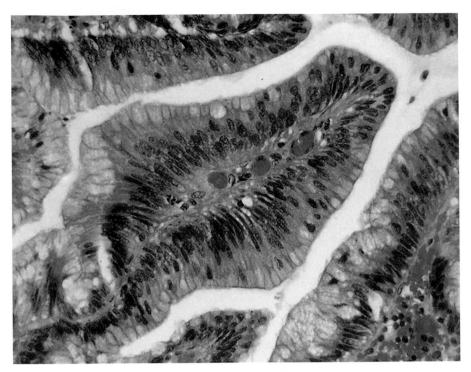

FIG. 8.7. Higher magnification of villous adenoma.

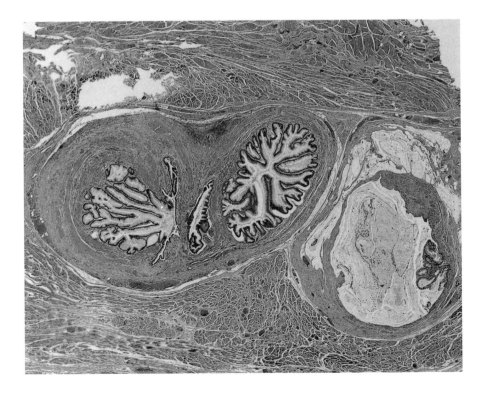

frequently present with villous adenoma, it necessitates thorough sampling of any lesion diagnosed by biopsy as villous adenoma.

In addition to in situ or invasive adenocarcinoma, urinary tract villous adenomas have been found in association with squamous cell carcinoma, flat in situ urothelial carcinoma, noninvasive papillary urothelial carcinoma, infiltrating urothelial carcinoma, and sarcomatoid urothelial carcinoma of the bladder. Associated urothelial carcinoma elements are not always discrete from the glandular villous adenomas, but often merge imperceptibly with them.

IN SITU ADENOCARCINOMA

Noninvasive papillary urothelial carcinomas may have glandlike lumina, which should be distinguished from in situ adenocarcinoma (efig 801). Chan and colleagues described a series of 19 cases of in situ adenocarcinoma of the bladder unaccompanied by infiltrating adenocarcinoma (13) (Figs. 8.9, 8.10) (efigs 799–824). In situ adenocarcinoma had a high incidence of association with urothelial carcinoma in situ (CIS) and specific subtypes of prognostically poor invasive carcinomas, such as small cell carcinoma and micropapillary urothelial carcinoma. These associations confirm that this disease is closely related to urothelial CIS.

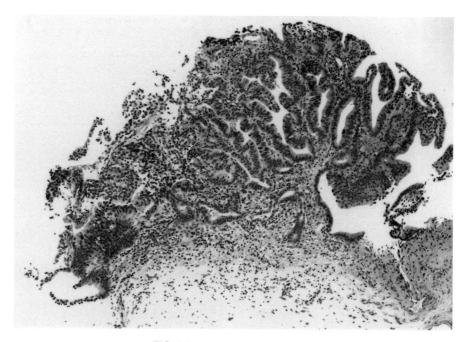

FIG. 8.9. In situ adenocarcinoma.

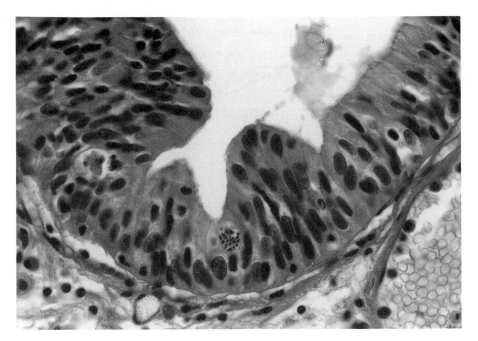

FIG. 8.10. Higher magnification of in situ adenocarcinoma.

INFILTRATING ADENOCARCINOMA

Primary pure adenocarcinomas of the bladder are rare, representing no more than 2.5% of all malignant vesical neoplasms. By definition, the tumor should be composed virtually entirely of glandular elements. As with other variants, they arise through a process of divergent (aberrant) differentiation in urothelial carcinoma (14–20). They constitute up to 90% of carcinomas associated with bladder extrophy. The tumor is also more frequently encountered in a setting of schistosomiasis. Shaaban and coworkers and El-Mekresh and colleagues reported series of 93 and 185 cases, respectively, of vesical adenocarcinoma arising in this setting (21,22). Adenocarcinomas can arise anywhere on the bladder surface, although a large percentage originates from the trigone and posterior wall. A major clinical difference between adenocarcinomas and the "usual" urothelial carcinomas is that two thirds of adenocarcinomas are single, discrete lesions, whereas usual urothelial carcinoma tends to be multifocal (23,24). Grossly, the tumors can be papillary, nodular, or flat and ulcerated. Microscopically, the tumor is most often composed of colonic-type glandular epithelium (enteric morphology) and contains abundant extracellular mucin (Figs. 8.11–8.13) (efigs 825–838). However, some tumors are highly cellular, are cytologically less well differentiated, and do not contain extracellular mucin. Regardless of histologic pattern, cystitis cystica et glandularis or surface glandular

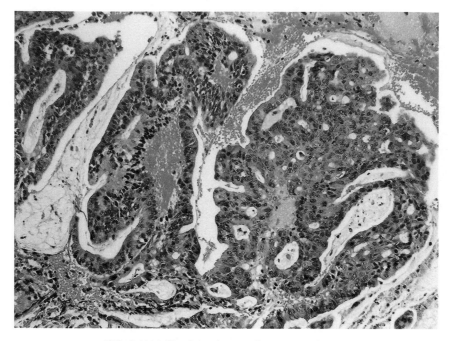

FIG. 8.11. Infiltrating adenocarcinoma, enteric type.

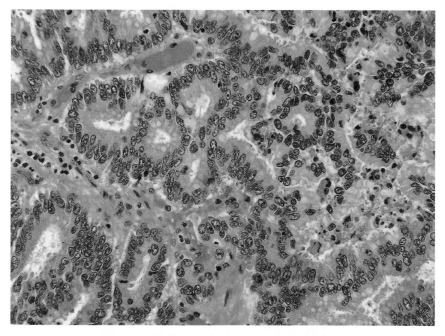

FIG. 8.12. Infiltrating adenocarcinoma, enteric type.

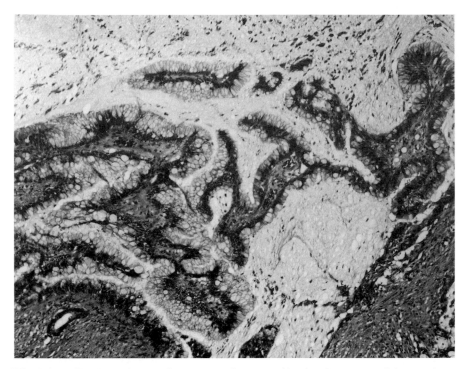

FIG. 8.13. Infiltrating adenocarcinoma, enteric type, with abundant extracellular mucinous secretions.

metaplasia is commonly present in the adjacent benign urothelium. Rarely, there may be associated villous adenoma of the bladder. Most adenocarcinomas have infiltrated deeply at the time of initial diagnosis, which most likely accounts for their poor prognosis. Stage for stage, they appear to have similar survival rates as usual urothelial carcinoma.

In the differential diagnosis, one must first consider the possibility of adenocarcinoma involving the bladder either by metastasis or direct invasion. Theoretically, it should be important to identify in situ carcinoma, although this is rarely possible on transurethral resection specimens due to ulceration of the overlying urothelium or to incomplete sampling. Secondary tumors such as colonic adenocarcinoma with invasion of the bladder wall may colonize the urothelium, mimicking in situ disease. Tumors that directly invade the bladder and mimic primary vesical adenocarcinoma include those arising in rectum, prostate, appendix, and endometrium (23–25). The only unequivocal way to establish such a tumor as a primary vesical neoplasm is to see a transition to usual urothelial carcinoma. For this reason, we routinely add the following disclaimer to our pathology report of the biopsy specimen: "We would accept as primary at this site if a metastasis or direct extension from an adjacent organ can be ruled out clinically." The treating clinician is in the best position to evaluate the patient and consider other primary sites.

Signet ring cell carcinoma of the bladder is a rare variant of adenocarcinoma with fewer than 70 cases reported in the English literature (26–30) (Figs. 8.14–8.17) (efigs 839–850). It is not uncommon to see signet ring cells within mucinous carcinomas, but we reserve the term *signet ring cell carcinoma* for those tumors composed almost entirely of signet ring or poorly differentiated round cells with intracytoplasmic mucin and without abundant extracellular mucin (diffuse-type adenocarcinoma). Except for their larger size, the cells are cytologically similar to mammary lobular carcinoma. Confirming origin in the bladder by finding CIS may be difficult, particularly on biopsy specimens. It is not unusual to find a dense layer of signet ring cells within the lamina propria directly below a denuded basement membrane (so-called cambium layer). These tumors tend to infiltrate the bladder wall diffusely, giving it an indurated and thickened quality similar to the "linitis plastica" seen in gastric signet ring cell carcinomas. The tumor also commonly infiltrates extensively throughout adjacent soft tissue, making primary resection for cure virtually impossible. Because of the advanced stage at presentation and poor prognosis, it is important to make the diagnosis on the TUR specimen, if possible. In the differential diagnosis, one must rule out direct extension, usually from a rectal carcinoma, or metastasis from stomach or lobular carcinoma of the breast or other organs (31).

In contrast, prostate carcinomas with a similar morphology are, with rare exception, composed of signet ring–like cells with empty clear vacuoles that do not usu-

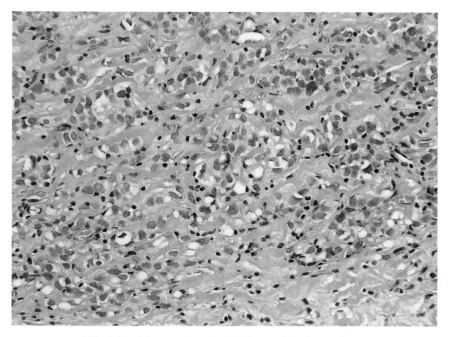

FIG. 8.14. Adenocarcinoma of bladder, signet ring cell type.

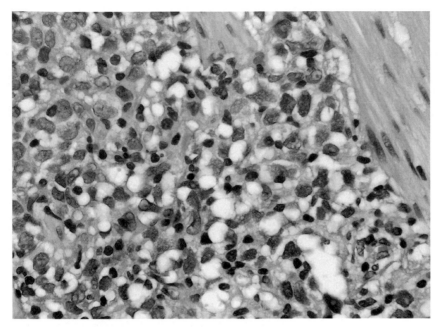

FIG. 8.15. Adenocarcinoma of bladder, signet ring cell type.

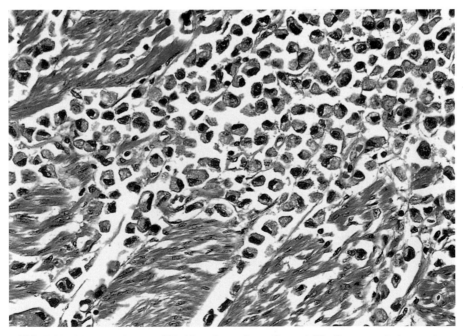

FIG. 8.16. Adenocarcinoma of bladder, signet ring cell type infiltrating muscularis propria.

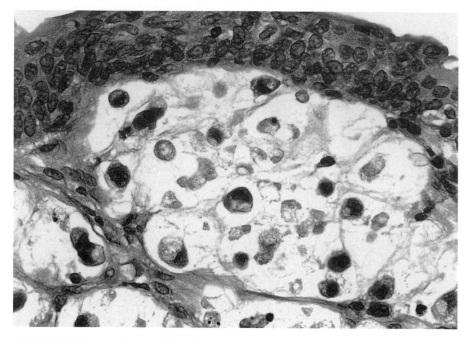

FIG. 8.17. Adenocarcinoma of bladder with extracellular mucin containing signet ring cells.

ally stain for mucin (see Chapter 13). Mucinous adenocarcinomas of the prostate typically reveal cords of epithelium and cribriform glands with bland cytology floating in mucin (32,33). The uniform cytology is typical of prostate cancer and differs from the greater anaplasia seen in bladder adenocarcinoma. The punched-out round lumina seen in the cribriform formations within prostate adenocarcinomas also helps to rule out bladder adenocarcinoma. Bladder adenocarcinomas, either as the sole component or admixed with urothelial elements, may in some cases show cross-reactive staining with antibodies to prostate-specific acid phosphatase (PSAP) (34). Although most bladder adenocarcinomas with PSAP positivity are focally positive as contrasted to the diffuse reactivity in prostate adenocarcinomas, careful consideration of the light microscopic appearance of the tumor is necessary to distinguish between an adenocarcinoma of the bladder and prostate.

URACHAL CARCINOMA

The urachus is a thick, tubelike structure formed in the embryo as the allantois involutes (efigs 851, 852). It extends from the bladder dome to the umbilicus. After birth, it becomes a fibrous cord called the *median umbilical ligament*. If remnants of the allantois (endoderm) remain within the ligament, they may develop into cysts as well as epithelial neoplasms. Such remnants have been found in 25% to 35% of bladders at the time of autopsy, usually in the dome but also along the anterior and rarely along the posterior bladder wall (35). The epithelial lining usually is urothelial, but in 33% of cases it undergoes glandular metaplasia. Neoplasms arising from the urachal remnant are usually adenocarcinomas and account for as much as 22% to 35% of vesical glandular neoplasms (36,37). Most adenocarcinomas have enteric features and are mucinous; some may have a signet ring cell component (38). Squamous cell, urothelial carcinomas, and anaplastic carcinomas also arise from the urachus (39). Rare cases of villous adenomas of the urachus have been reported, sometimes associated with mucosuria, suggesting communication with the bladder lumen (40).

Because the urachus is usually found along the free surface of the bladder, urachal carcinomas are frequently amenable to partial cystectomy. Because the entire length of the median umbilical ligament may harbor urachal remnants that may develop carcinoma synchronously or metachronously, the surgery of choice should include en bloc resection of the entire length of the ligament including the umbilicus (41). The bladder is usually only partially resected owing to the unifocality of the tumor.

Several criteria must be met to establish the diagnosis of urachal carcinoma. The bladder involvement by tumor should be localized to an area usually at or near the dome in relation to the medial umbilical ligament. The overlying bladder urothelium may be ulcerated but no in situ carcinoma or glandular metaplasia should be present (other than cystitis glandularis). Often, this issue is difficult to address because the overlying epithelium is ulcerated or previously biopsied. Rarely, the urachal tumor communicates directly with the bladder surface. Occasionally, urachal remnants are found, characterized by cystic structures of variable size lined by urothelium or benign glandular epithelium. A metastatic tumor should be ruled out clinically.

The differential diagnosis includes metastatic adenocarcinoma and primary adenocarcinoma arising from the bladder surface. The latter is usually associated with an intraluminal mass and the diagnosis is established by finding in situ carcinoma or extensive glandular metaplasia of the adjacent urothelium. Because these features are rarely seen on a transurethral resection of bladder tumor (TURBT) specimen of an ulcerated lesion, we include the following note in the pathology report of any solitary glandular lesion involving the dome of the bladder: "We would accept as primary at this site, including the possibility of urachal origin, if a metastasis or direct extension from an adjacent organ has been ruled out." Once again, the urologist is in the best position to make this determination.

CARCINOMAS WITH DIVERGENT (ABERRANT) DIFFERENTIATION

Urothelial carcinomas, particularly high-grade tumors, may show divergent differentiation (Fig. 8.18) (efigs 853–861). Urothelial carcinomas with true glandular differentiation must be distinguished from urothelial carcinomas with glandlike lumina. The latter is not uncommon and represents microcystic change

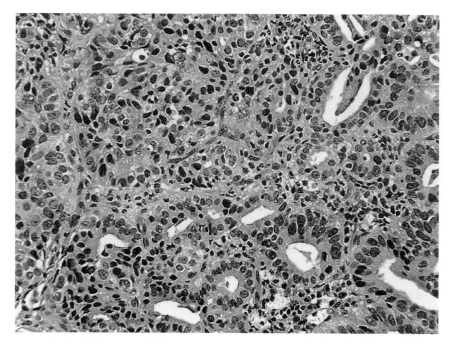

FIG. 8.18. Urothelial carcinoma with glandular differentiation.

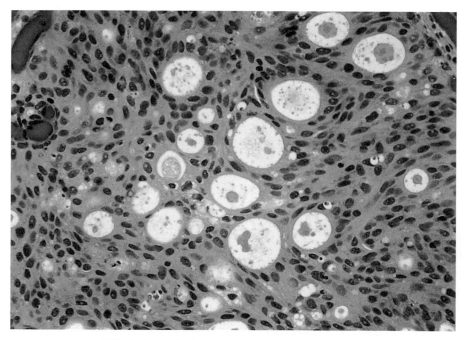

FIG. 8.19. Urothelial carcinoma with glandlike lumina.

within an otherwise typical urothelial carcinoma (Fig. 8.19). Although these spaces may contain mucin, they differ from urothelial carcinoma admixed with a well-defined adenocarcinoma component. Divergent differentiation is seen primarily in invasive urothelial tumors but may occasionally be present with in situ disease. The entire spectrum of histologic variants may be encountered accompanying "usual" urothelial carcinoma, mostly in cases of high-grade and high-stage disease. In a series of 300 consecutive cystectomies performed at Memorial Sloan-Kettering Cancer Center, 27% of cancer-bearing specimens contained some form of divergent differentiation. The incidence would be lower in TURBT specimens and in different types of medical institutions. At Memorial, where patients usually fall into a high-risk category, the incidence can be as high as 7%. When divergent differentiation is seen together with usual urothelial carcinoma, the pathologist should use the terminology of *urothelial carcinoma with* ____ *differentiation*, inserting in the space the type of differentiation observed.

CLEAR CELL ADENOCARCINOMA

Clear cell adenocarcinoma may arise in the bladder. Morphologically these neoplasms have one or more of the three typical features seen in clear cell carcinomas of the female genital tract, including tubulocystic, papillary, and diffuse patterns (Figs. 8.20–8.23) (efigs 862–870). These tumors initially were thought

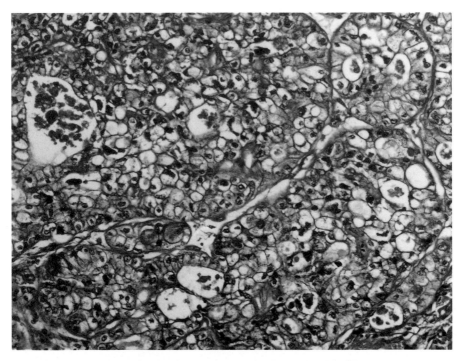

FIG. 8.20. Clear cell (mesonephric) adenocarcinoma.

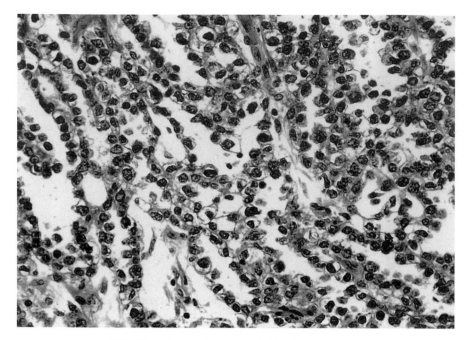

FIG. 8.21. Clear cell (mesonephric) adenocarcinoma.

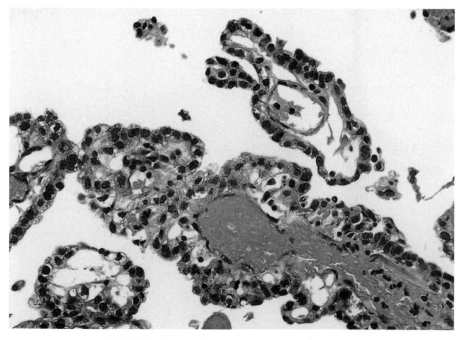

FIG. 8.22. Clear cell (mesonephric) adenocarcinoma.

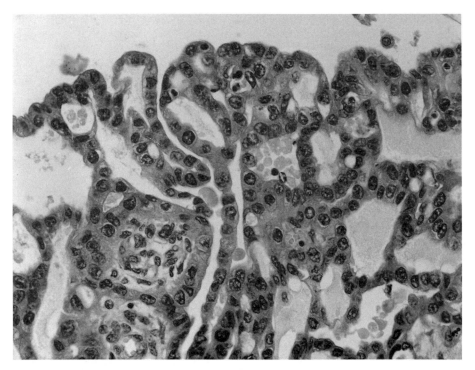

FIG. 8.23. Area of clear cell (mesonephric) adenocarcinoma which on a small biopsy could be difficult to distinguish from nephrogenic adenoma.

to arise from mesonephric rests in the trigone area, but we now believe that they may arise through a process of metaplasia of the surface urothelium or from müllerian rests or müllerianosis (42–45). In a series of 13 cases, Oliva and co-workers found that four were likely of müllerian origin while the remaining nine could have arisen from the urothelium. Interestingly, this series included 11 females and 2 males. This strong female predominance is rare for urothelial tumors and suggests that müllerian origin may account for an even larger percent of these cases. Immunohistochemical studies are not useful in establishing histogenesis (45).

The morphologic features are characteristic but vary between tumors because more than one pattern may be seen. Tubules and papillae are generally lined by flat, cuboidal, or, rarely, columnar cells. Sheetlike growth and cystic architecture may also be present. Clear cells are abundant in most tumors, although virtually all tumors also have cells with abundant eosinophilic cytoplasm as well. Hobnail cells are present in most tumors but are conspicuous in the minority. Nuclear atypia is moderate to severe, although rare cases with bland cytology have been described. Mitotic activity is present but may be quite variable. Necrosis may be evident. Clear cell adenocarcinomas are high-grade, infiltrating carcinomas with frequent mitoses, nuclear pleomorphism, and areas of solid growth, all of which is absent in nephrogenic adenoma (metaplasia). Direct extension from an adjacent pelvic organ must also be ruled out clinically.

ENDOMETRIOSIS, ENDOCERVICOSIS, AND MÜLLERIANOSIS

Whereas most glandular lesions involving the urinary bladder arise through a process of metaplasia of the surface urothelium, that is not the case with these types of lesions. Genitourinary involvement by endometriosis occurs in 1% to 2% of cases. More than 200 cases of vesical endometriosis have been described, making the urinary bladder the most common site of involvement within the urinary tract (46–48). Classically, it affects women between the second and fifth decade of life but may rarely be seen in postmenopausal women receiving exogenous estrogen (49). Interestingly, rare cases of vesical endometriosis have been described in males with prostate carcinoma who were receiving exogenous estrogen therapy (50,51). The occurrence in males is intriguing and most likely represents activation of müllerian rests by exogenous estrogens. Clinically, patients present with urgency, frequency, suprapubic pain, and rarely hematuria. A mass is frequently apparent either by palpation or cystoscopic examination (52,53). The lesion may reside in the superficial or deep layers of the vesical wall or in the adjacent perivesical soft tissue so that a simple transurethral biopsy may not

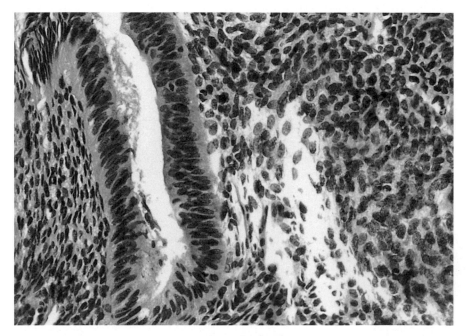

FIG. 8.24. Endometriosis.

always provide diagnostic tissue. Microscopically, the lesion resembles endometriosis elsewhere; endometrium-like glandular epithelium is present in association with endometrial stromal cells and recent or old hemorrhage (Fig. 8.24) (efigs 871, 872). Rarely, one finds only glands or stroma. In the former case, the differential diagnosis must include infiltrating adenocarcinoma, from which it is distinguished by its recognizable growth pattern characteristics and by the uniform and orderly glands of endometriosis. Endometriosis may involve the lower third of the ureter where it may produce obstructive symptoms. Endometriosis involving the urethra is extremely rare.

Endocervicosis of the urinary bladder is a rare condition first described as a distinct entity by Clement and Young in 1992 (54). It is seen in women of child-bearing age who present with a mass in the posterior wall or posterior dome, usually associated with suprapubic pain, frequency, and dysuria. It is thought to arise from müllerian rests and is characterized by extensive involvement of the bladder wall by benign or mildly atypical, columnar, mucin-secreting endocer-vical-like glands (Figs. 8.25–8.28) (efigs 872–883). Extravasation of mucin is present in all cases secondary to gland rupture. Because endocervicosis of the bladder is commonly located deep within the viscus and is associated with a mass, it must be distinguished from an invasive carcinoma clinically and from

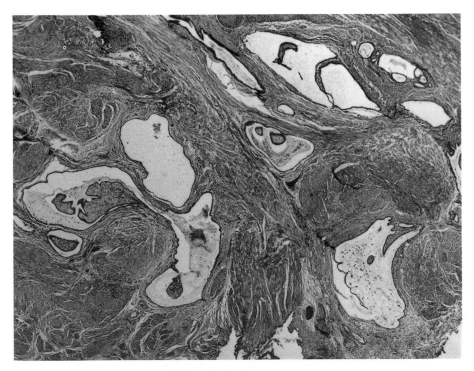

FIG. 8.25. Endocervicosis.

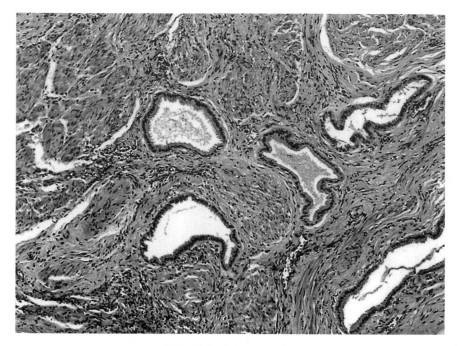

FIG. 8.26. Endocervicosis.

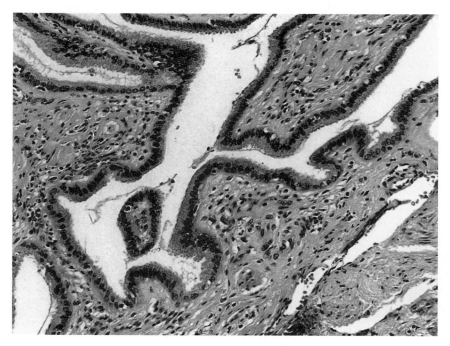

FIG. 8.27. Endocervicosis.

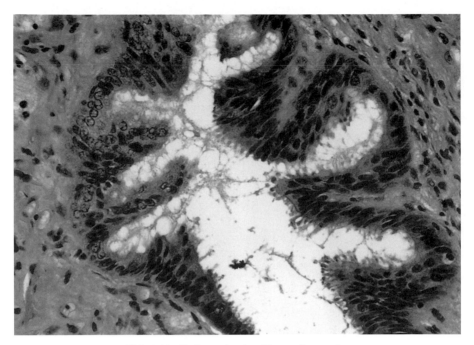

FIG. 8.28. Endocervicosis with reactive atypia.

adenocarcinoma morphologically (55). In contrast to adenocarcinoma, there is no or at most minimal atypia, no mitotic figures, and no tissue reaction.

In 1996, Clement and Young described müllerianosis of the urinary bladder (56). These rare lesions occur in the same clinical setting as endocervicosis, differing only in that the lesion may contain other benign müllerian-type components including endometrial or tubal epithelium. Once again, care must be taken not to confuse such lesions with adenocarcinoma (56–58).

NEPHROGENIC ADENOMA (METAPLASIA)

The other lesion that may mimic adenocarcinoma is nephrogenic adenoma (nephrogenic metaplasia) (Figs. 8.29–8.32) (Color Plates 9, 10) (efigs 884–895). Nephrogenic adenomas usually arise in the setting of prior urothelial injury, such as past surgery (60%), calculi (14%), or trauma (9%) (59). Eight percent have a history of renal transplantation. Approximately two thirds of individuals affected with nephrogenic adenomas are male, and in one third the lesion is found when patients are younger than 30 years of age. Nephrogenic adenomas appear as papillary, polypoid, hyperplastic, fungating, friable, or velvety lesions. They are located throughout the bladder, although they are rarely found on the anterior wall. Eighty percent are localized to the bladder, with 12% seen in the urethra and 8% in the ureter. Most nephrogenic adenomas measure less than 1 cm,

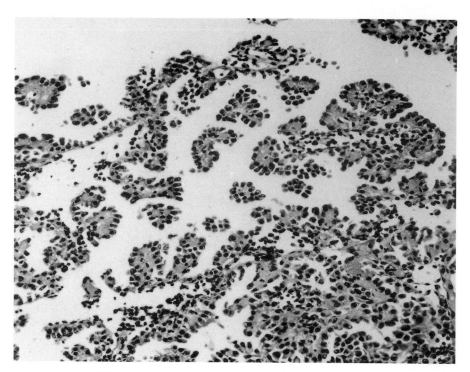

FIG. 8.29. Nephrogenic adenoma with papillary formation.

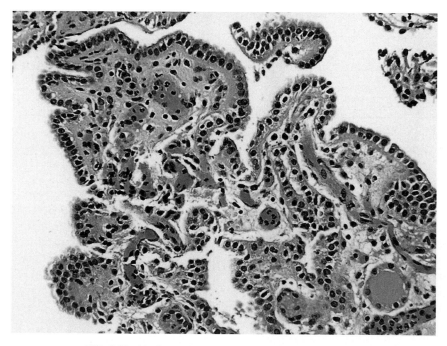

FIG. 8.30. Nephrogenic adenoma with papillary formation.

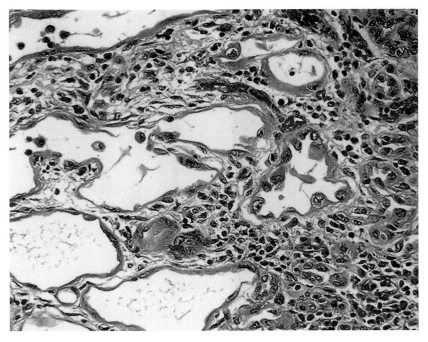

FIG. 8.31. Nephrogenic adenoma with structures resembling vessels and hobnail atypia.

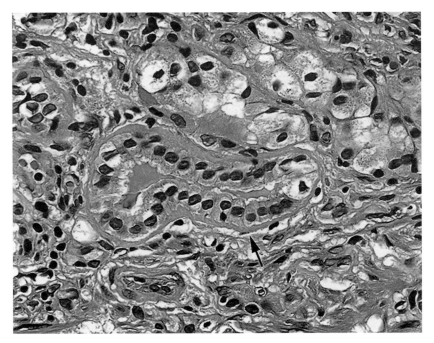

FIG. 8.32. Nephrogenic adenoma. Note hyaline basement membrane-like material (*arrow*).

although they may attain dimensions as large as 7 cm. In 18% of cases, multiple lesions are identified.

Nephrogenic adenomas have a broad histologic spectrum (60). A common pattern consists of tubules lined by low columnar to cuboidal epithelium. Nuclear atypia is virtually absent with mitoses being either absent or rare, although prominent nucleoli may be visualized. Nuclear atypia, when present, appears degenerative. Nuclei are enlarged and hyperchromatic, yet have a smudged indistinct chromatin pattern. These atypical nuclei often reside in cells with an endothelial or hobnail appearance lining vascular-like dilated tubules. Cystic tubules may contain colloid-like eosinophilic or basophilic secretions. Uncommonly, tubules are lined by either more columnar cells with pale cytoplasm or signet appearing cells; clear cells are rare and glycogen is usually absent. Nephrogenic adenomas may also be papillary, usually lined by low cuboidal cells with scant cytoplasm or, on occasion, by oxyphilic cells. The tubules are often surrounded by a thickened and hyalinized basement membrane and do not incite a stromal response; the stroma may be edematous. A focal solid growth pattern may be present although it is frequently associated with other patterns. Variable numbers of acute and chronic inflammatory cells are commonplace within the bladder wall. In contrast to adenocarcinoma, nephrogenic adenomas lack conspicuous solid growth patterns, mitotic activity, and prominent cytologic atypia, and they are not typically large, deeply invasive tumors. We have seen rare cases of nephrogenic adenomas focally involve the superficial aspects of the muscularis propria. Nephrogenic adenoma may be weakly immunoreactive for prostate-specific antigen or PSAP as a further pitfall in the differential diagnosis with adenocarcinoma of the prostate.

Nephrogenic adenoma is thought to be due to an inflammatory insult or local injury (61–64). It was originally described in the trigone and given its name because it was thought to arise from mesonephric rests. Mazal and coworkers studied cases of nephrogenic adenoma in kidney transplant recipients (65). Based on FISH and lectin studies, they concluded that these lesions were derived from shed tubular cells originating from the transplanted kidney rather than from a metaplastic process. We remain unconvinced that this process is the genesis of most cases of nephrogenic adenoma, at least in the general population.

REFERENCES

1. Mostofi FK. Potentialities of bladder epithelium. *J Urol* 1954;71:705–714.
2. Davies G, Castro JE. Cystitis glandularis. *Urology* 1977;10:128–129.
3. Young RH, Bostwick DG. Florid cystitis glandularis of intestinal type with mucin extravasation: a mimic of adenocarcinoma. *Am J Surg Pathol* 1996;20:1462–1468.
4. Jacobs LB, Brooks JD, Epstein JI. Differentiation of colonic metaplasia from adenocarcinoma of urinary bladder. *Hum Pathol* 1997;28:1152–1157.
5. Corica FA, Husmann DA, Churchill BM, et al: Intestinal metaplasia is not a strong risk factor for bladder cancer: study of 53 cases with long-term follow up. *Urology* 1997;50:427–431.
6. Engel RM, Wilkson HA. Bladder extrophy. *J Urol* 1970;104:699–704.
7. Nielsen K, Nielson KK. Adenocarcinoma in extrophy of the bladder—the last case in Scandinavia? A case report and review of literature. *J Urol* 1983;130:1180–1182.

8. Assor D. A villous tumor of the bladder. *J Urol* 1978;119:287–288.
9. Miller DC, Gang DL, Gauris V, et al. Villous adenoma of the bladder: a morphologic or biologic entity? *Am J Clin Pathol* 1983;79:728–731.
10. Newman J, Antonakopoulos GN. Widespread mucus metaplasia of the urinary bladder with nephrogenic adenoma. *Arch Pathol Lab Med* 1985;109:560–563.
11. Liang C, Montironi R, Bostwick DG. Villous adenoma of the urinary tract: a report of 23 cases, including 8 with coexistent adenocarcinoma. *Am J Surg Pathol* 1999;23:764–771.
12. Seibel J, Prasad S, Weiss RE, et al. Villous adenoma of the urinary tract: a lesion frequently associated with malignancy. *Hum Pathol* 2002;33:236–241.
13. Chan TY, Epstein JI. In situ adenocarcinoma of the bladder. *Am J Surg Pathol* 2001;25:892–899.
14. Wheeler JD, Hill WT. Adenocarcinoma involving the urinary bladder. *Cancer* 1954;7:119–135.
15. Mostofi FK, Thomson RV, Dean AL. Mucous adenocarcinoma of the urinary bladder. *Cancer* 1955;8:741–758.
16. Nocks BN, Heney NM, Daly JJ. Primary adenocarcinoma of urinary bladder. *Urology* 1983;21:26–29.
17. Anderstrom C, Johansson SL, von Schultz L. Primary adenocarcinoma of the urinary bladder: a clinicopathologic and prognostic study. *Cancer* 1983;52:1273–1282.
18. Grignon DJ, Ro JY, Ayala AG, et al. Primary adenocarcinoma of the urinary bladder: a clinicopathologic analysis of 72 cases. *Cancer* 1991;67:2165–2172.
19. Jones WA, Gibbons RP, Correa RJ, et al. Primary adenocarcinoma of the bladder. *Urology* 1980;15:119–122.
20. Malek RS, Rosen JS, O'Dea MJ. Adenocarcinoma of the bladder. *Urology* 1983;20:357–359.
21. Shaaban AA, Elbaz MA, Tribukait. Primary nonurachal adenocarcinoma in the bilharzial urinary bladder: deoxyribonucleic acid flow cytometric and morphologic characterization in 93 cases. *Urol* 1998;51:469–476.
22. El-Mekresh MM, El-Baz MA, Abol-Enein H, et al. Primary adenocarcinoma of the urinary bladder: a report of 185 cases. *Br J Urol* 1998;82:206–212.
23. Dean AL, Mostofi FK, Thompson RV. A restudy of the first fourteen hundred tumors in the bladder tumor registry. *J Urol* 1954;71:571–590.
24. Melicow MM. Tumors of the urinary bladder. A clinicopathological analysis of over 2,500 specimens and autopsies. *J Urol* 1955;74:498–521.
25. Bischoff W, Bohn N. Adenocarcinoma of the appendix penetrating the bladder. *J Urol* 1980;123:123–126.
26. Braun EV, Ali M, Fayemi O, et al. Primary signet-ring cell carcinoma of the urinary bladder: review of the literature and report of a case. *Cancer* 1981;47:1430–1435.
27. Poore TE, Egbert B, Jahnke R, et al. Signet ring cell adenocarcinoma of the bladder: linitis plastica variant. *Arch Pathol Lab Med* 1981;105:203–204.
28. Choi H, Lamb S, Pintar K, et al. Primary signet-ring cell carcinoma of the urinary bladder. *Cancer* 1984;53:1985–1990.
29. Bernstein SA, Reuter VE, Carroll PR, et al. Primary signet ring cell carcinoma of the urinary bladder. *Urology* 1988;31:432–436.
30. Grignon DJ, Ro JY, Ayala AG, et al. Primary signet ring cell carcinoma of the urinary bladder. *Am J Clin Pathol* 1991;95:13–20.
31. Pontes JE, Oldford JR. Metastatic breast carcinoma to the bladder. *J Urol* 1970;104:839–842.
32. Epstein JI, Lieberman PH. Mucinous adenocarcinoma of the prostate gland. *Am J Surg Pathol* 1985;9:299–308.
33. Ro JY, Grignon DJ, Ayala AG, et al. Mucinous adenocarcinoma of the prostate: histochemical and immunohistochemical studies. *Hum Pathol* 1990;21:593–600.
34. Epstein JI, Kuhajda FP, Lieberman PH. Prostate-specific acid phosphatase immunoreactivity in adenocarcinomas of the urinary bladder. *Hum Pathol* 1986;17:939–942.
35. Schubert GE, Paukovic MB, Bethke-Bedurftig BA. Tubular urachal remnants in adult bladders. *J Urol* 1982;127:40–42.
36. Johnson DE, Hodge GB, Abdul-Karim FW, et al. Urachal carcinoma. *Urology* 1985;26:218–221.
37. Jakse G, Schneider HM, Jacobi GH. Urachal signet-ring cell carcinoma, a rare variant of vesical adenocarcinoma: incidence and pathological criteria. *J Urol* 1978;120:764–766.
38. Alonso-Gorrea M, Mompo-Sanchis JA, Jorda-Cuevas M, et al. Signet ring cell adenocarcinoma of the urachus. *Eur Urol* 1985;11:282–284.
39. Ghazizadeh M, Yamamoto S, Kurokawa K. Clinical features of urachal carcinoma in Japan: review of 157 patients. *Urol Res* 1983;11:235–238.

40. Eble JN, Hull MT, Rowland RG, et al. Villous adenoma of the urachus with mucosuria: a light and electron microscopic study. *J Urol* 1986;135:1240–1244.
41. Hayman J. Carcinoma of the urachus. *Pathology* 1984;16:167–171.
42. Skor AB, Warren MM. Mesonephric adenocarcinoma of the bladder. *Urol* 1977;10:64–65.
43. Schultz RE, Block MJ, Tomaszewski JE, et al. Mesonephric adenocarcinoma of the bladder. *J Urol* 1984;132:263–265.
44. Young RH, Scully RE. Clear cell adenocarcinoma of the bladder and urethra: a report of three cases and review of the literature. *Am J Surg Pathol* 1985;9:816–826.
45. Oliva E, Amin MB, Jimenez R, et al. Clear cell carcinoma of the urinary bladder. A report and comparison of four tumors of Müllerian origin and nine of probable urothelial origin with discussion of histogenesis and diagnostic problems. *Am J Surg Pathol* 2002;26:190–197.
46. Nixon WCW. Endometriosis of the bladder. *Lancet* 1940;1:405–406.
47. Fein RL, Horton BF. Vesical endometriosis: a case report and review of the literature. *J Urol* 1966;95:45–50.
48. Lichtenfeld FR, McCauley RT, Staples PP. Endometriosis involving the urinary tract. A collective review. *Obstet Gynecol* 1961;17:762–768.
49. Stewart WW, Ireland GW. Vesical endometriosis in a postmenopausal woman: a case report. *J Urol* 1977;118:480–481.
50. Pinkert TC, Catlow CE, Straus R. Endometriosis of the urinary bladder in a man with prostatic carcinoma. *Cancer* 1979;43:1562–1567.
51. Randolph Schrodt G, Alcorn MO, Ibanez J. Endometriosis of the male urinary system: a case report. *J Urol* 1980;124:722–723.
52. Lenaine WO, Admundsen CL, McGuire EJ. Bladder endometriosis: conservative management. *J Urol* 2000;163:1814–1817.
53. Comiter CV. Endometriosis of the urinary tract. *Urol Clin North Am* 2002;29:625–635.
54. Clement PB, Young RH. Endocervicosis of the urinary bladder. A report of six cases of a benign müllerian lesion that may mimic adenocarcinoma. *Am J Surg Pathol* 1992;16:533–542.
55. Julié C, Boyé K, Desgrippes A, et al. Endocervicosis of the urinary bladder. Immunohistochemical comparative study between a new case and normal uterine endocervices. *Pathol Res Pract* 2002;198:115–198.
56. Young RH, Clement PB. Müllerianosis of the urinary bladder. *Mod Pathol* 1996;9:731–737.
57. Kim HJ, Lee TJ, Kim MK, et al. Müllerianosis of the urinary bladder, endocervicosis type: a case report. *J Korean Med Sci* 2001;16:123–126.
58. Donné C, Vidal M, Buttin X, et al. Müllerianosis of the urinary bladder: clinical and immunohistochemical findings. *Histopathology* 1998;33:284–285.
59. Baghavan BS, Tiamson EM, Wenk RE, et al. Nephrogenic adenoma of the urinary bladder and urethra. *Human Pathol* 1981;12:907–916.
60. Allen CH, Epstein JI. Nephrogenic adenoma of the prostatic urethra: a mimicker of prostate adenocarcinoma. *Am J Surg Pathol* 2001;25:802–808.
61. Stilment MM, Sivoky MB. Nephrogenic adenoma associated with intravesical bacillus Calmette-Guerin treatment: a report of two cases. *J Urol* 1986;135:359–361.
62. Navarre RJ, Loening SA, Narayana A. Nephrogenic adenoma: a report of nine cases and review of the literature. *J Urol* 1982;127:775–779.
63. Molland EA, Trott PA, Paris MI, et al. Nephrogenic adenoma: a form of adenomatous metaplasia of the bladder. A clinical and electron microscopical study. *Br J Urol* 1976;48:453–462.
64. Ford TF, Watson GM, Cameron KM. Adenomatous metaplasia (nephrogenic adenoma) of urothelium: an analysis of 70 cases. *Br J Urol* 1985;57:427–433.
65. Mazal PR, Schaufler R, Altenhuber-Muller R, et al. *N Engl J Med* 2002;347:684–686.

9

Squamous Lesions

SQUAMOUS METAPLASIA

Squamous metaplasia, particularly in the area of the trigone is a common finding in women (efigs 68–74) (see Chapter 1). It is likely that trigonal squamous metaplasia in women indeed represents a normal histologic variant unassociated with local injury. Under other conditions, the metaplastic squamous epithelium undergoes keratinization and may exhibit parakeratosis, hyperkeratosis, and even acquire a granular layer (efigs 75, 76) (see Chapter 1). This metaplastic epithelium is not preneoplastic per se, but under some circumstances it may lead to squamous carcinoma (1). This is the sequence of events, for example, in patients with long-standing schistosomiasis of the urinary bladder or, in the case of squamous carcinoma, arising in bladder diverticula (2–4). In these cases it may be possible to observe keratinizing squamous metaplasia adjacent to in situ and invasive squamous carcinoma. The pathologist is obligated to mention the presence and extent of keratinizing squamous metaplasia in a transurethral biopsy specimen. Khan and colleagues described their experience with 34 patients with histologically proven keratinizing squamous metaplasia. Although the extent of involvement was important, the authors concluded that it represented a significant risk factor for the development of subsequent carcinoma as well as other complications such as bladder contracture and obstruction (5). Keratinizing squamous metaplasia may be seen in urothelium of patients with high-grade urothelial carcinoma and is an expression of divergent differentiation in the surface component of the urothelium.

CONDYLOMA

Condyloma acuminata are common sexually transmitted benign tumors caused by a human papillomavirus (PPV) (Figs. 9.1, 9.2) (efigs 896–904). They occur most frequently on mucocutaneous surfaces of the external genitalia, perineum, and anus but extension into the urethra is not uncommon, occurring in up to 20% of cases. On rare occasions, they may involve the bladder or even the ureters (6–8). Condyloma affecting the bladder exclusively is rare. These lesions

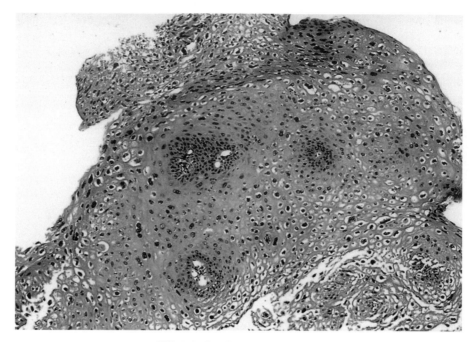

FIG. 9.1. Condyloma acuminatum.

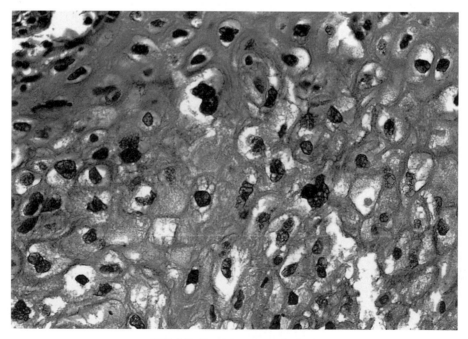

FIG. 9.2. Condyloma acuminatum.

may be discrete, but there is a tendency toward diffuse involvement. Macroscopically the lesions are smooth, pink-tan, and papillary. If there is diffuse involvement, the urothelial surface takes on a velvety appearance. Microscopically the lesions are characterized by papillary fronds lined by hyperplastic, metaplastic squamous epithelium, which may be hyperkeratotic. Typically, many of the epithelial cells have a perinuclear halo, an empty or clear area of the cytoplasm surrounding an eccentrically placed, hyperchromatic, irregular nucleus. Binucleate forms are common. These cells have been given the descriptive name of *koilocytes*. Immunohistochemical stains using antipapillomavirus antibodies or in situ hybridization for HPV identifies the cells containing the virus. They may also be cultured for positive identification. These cells commonly overexpress p53 nuclear protein by immunohistochemistry.

Condylomata of the urinary tract may cause irritative symptoms and hematuria. Discrete lesions are managed by transurethral resection, but diffuse disease usually necessitates more radical surgery. One also must be aware of the risk of malignant transformation in condylomata and the development of verrucous carcinoma (9).

SQUAMOUS CELL CARCINOMA

The diagnosis of squamous cell carcinoma should be reserved for those tumors that are purely or almost entirely keratin forming (Fig. 9.3) (efigs

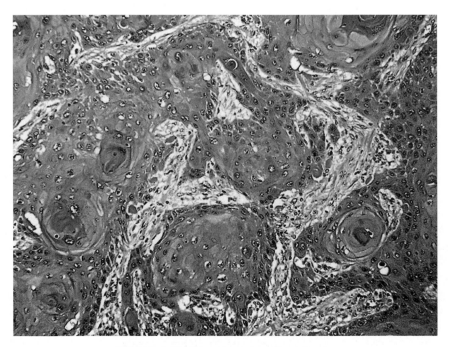

FIG. 9.3. Infiltrating squamous cell carcinoma.

905–909). For urothelial tumors with variable amounts of squamous differentiation, the term *urothelial carcinoma with squamous differentiation* should be used [see Chapter 8 for important general concepts regarding divergent (aberrant) differentiation]. Squamous carcinomas constitute 2% to 7% of urothelial cancers, except in the Middle East.

Along the Nile Valley, as a consequence of the endemic nature of schistosomiasis, squamous carcinomas are the most common form of cancer (2,10,11) (see Chapter 10). Nitrates in the urine, particularly present in individuals living in agricultural areas where nitrate fertilizers are used liberally, may be reduced to carcinogenic nitrosamines as a result of secondary bacterial infection. Between 60% and 90% of carcinomas associated with urinary schistosomiasis are squamous cell carcinomas, with 5% to 15% being adenocarcinomas and the rest urothelial carcinomas. The tumors typically are nodular fungating masses occupying the dome or posterolateral walls of the bladder. Almost half of the squamous cell carcinomas associated with urinary schistosomiasis are well differentiated and have a fairly good prognosis. The reported 5-year disease-free survival after radical cystectomy for schistosomal associated carcinoma is approximately 48%. Factors affecting survival include tumor stage, grade, and lymph node involvement. Specific tumor type does not appear to influence outcome. Treatment is by radical cystoprostatectomy or radical cystectomy with apparently little added benefit from radiation or chemotherapy. Godwin and colleagues reviewed a series of 160 cases of bladder carcinoma seen at King Faisal Hospital in Saudi Arabia (2). Of these, approximately one third were associated with schistosomiasis, 72% of which had squamous cell carcinoma. Whereas 41% of patients in the nonschistosomiasis group presented with noninvasive disease or infiltration limited to the lamina propria, only 8% of schistosomal related tumors presented at these early stages.

Squamous carcinomas in general tend to be sessile, ulcerated, and infiltrative at the time of diagnosis. The histologic hallmarks of keratin-pearl formation, intercellular bridges, and keratotic cellular debris are those of squamous carcinoma at any site. Except the verrucous variant, most of these carcinomas are moderately or poorly differentiated and more deeply invasive at the time of diagnosis than the majority of urothelial carcinomas. Their generally poor prognosis can be attributed to the typically advanced stage at diagnosis, but stage for stage, prognosis is similar for squamous and usual type of urothelial carcinoma (11).

Squamous carcinoma of the urothelial tract is thought to arise through a process of metaplasia of the urothelium. A large percentage of patients with squamous cell carcinoma have squamous metaplasia of the adjacent urothelium. Many have a history of severe, long-term, chronic inflammation associated with stones, chronic infection, bilharziasis, and, in a few, prior systemic chemotherapy with cyclophosphamide (12).

It is rare for squamous carcinoma in situ to be diagnosed in the absence of an invasive component (Figs. 9.4, 9.5) (efigs 174–177, 910–913). If such a diagnosis is rendered, the urologist should be counseled to either rebiopsy or closely

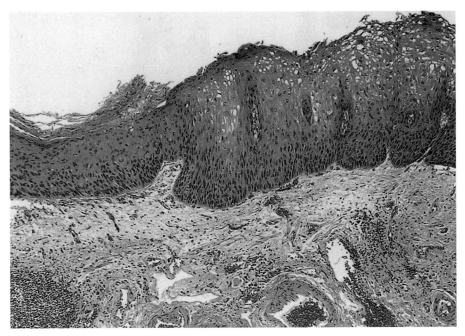

FIG. 9.4. In situ squamous cell carcinoma.

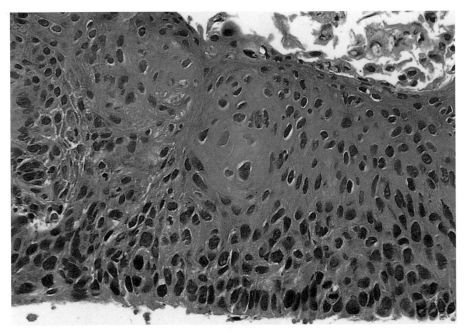

FIG. 9.5. Higher magnification of Figure 9.4 showing in situ squamous cell carcinoma.

follow up the patient for unsampled or subsequent development of invasive squamous carcinoma, respectively.

SQUAMOUS PAPILLOMA

In 2000, Cheng and colleagues described a series of seven cases of squamous papilloma, five occurring in the urinary bladder and the others in the urethra (13) (Fig. 9.6) (efig 914). These lesions were characterized by a proliferation of mature and benign-appearing squamous epithelium surrounding a central fibrovascular core. Koilocytes were not present, the cells did not show high levels of nuclear p53 overexpression, and in situ hybridization for HPV was negative in all cases. Most of the patients were women and none had history of genital, perianal, or perineal condyloma. It must be emphasized that these lesions are very rare compared with condylomata. The relationship of squamous papilloma to the development of carcinoma is unknown.

VERRUCOUS CARCINOMA

Verrucous carcinoma is a rare variant of infiltrating squamous carcinoma more commonly seen in the oral cavity, anus, or genital areas (Figs. 9.7, 9.8) (efigs 915–920). It is a very low-grade, orderly carcinoma that is clinically indo-

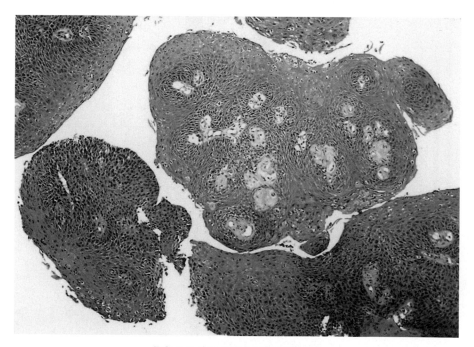

FIG. 9.6. Squamous cell papilloma.

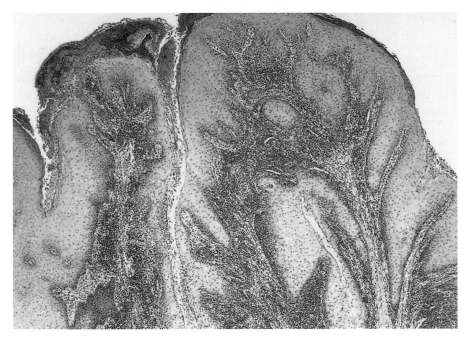

FIG. 9.7. Verrucous carcinoma.

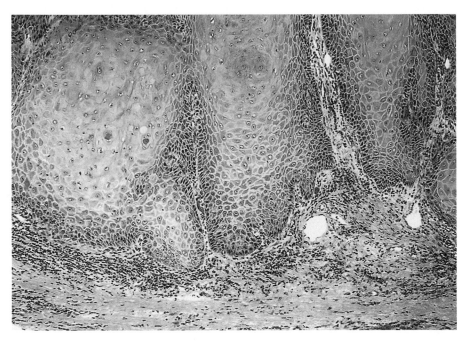

FIG. 9.8. Base of verrucous carcinoma with pushing invasive border.

lent, characterized by local invasion by broad-pushing tongues of bland squamous epithelium. The diagnosis of cancer is based on the finding that the squamous downgrowth of epithelium is too deep to represent an artifact of sectioning, verrucous hyperplasia, or pseudoepitheliomatous hyperplasia and hence must represent invasion (efigs 921–922). Few cases involving the bladder have been reported, usually in association with schistosomiasis or condyloma acuminatum (10,14–17). Because transurethral resection specimens are rarely well oriented, it may be difficult to diagnose verrucous carcinoma on transurethral resection specimens, unless there is ample characteristic tumor or tumor is seen in the muscularis propria.

REFERENCES

 1. Tannenbaum M. Inflammatory proliferative lesion of the urinary bladder: squamous metaplasia. *Urology* 1976;7:428–429.
 2. Godwin JT, Hanash K. Pathology of bilharzial bladder cancer. In: Bladder cancer, part A: pathology, diagnosis and surgery. New York: Alan R. Liss, 1984:95–143.
 3. Zahran MM, Kamel M, Mooro H, et al. Bilharziasis of urinary bladder and ureter: comparative histopathologic study. *Urology* 1976;8:73–79.
 4. Kertsschmer HL. Diverticula of the urinary bladder. A clinical study of 236 cases. *Surg Gynecol Obstet* 1940;71:491–503.
 5. Khan MS, Thornhill JA, Gaffney E, et al. Keratinizing squamous metaplasia of the bladder: natural history and rationalization of management based on review of 54 years' experience. *Eur Urol* 2002;42:469–474.
 6. Bissada NK, Cole AT, Fried FA. Extensive condyloma acuminata of the entire male urethra and the bladder. *J Urol* 1974;112:201–203.
 7. DeBenedictis TJ, Marmar JL, Praiss DE. Intraurethral condyloma acuminata: management and review of the literature. *J Urol* 1977;118:767–769.
 8. Keating MA, Young RH, Carr CP, et al. Condyloma acuminatum of the bladder and ureter: case report and review of the literature. *J Urol* 1985;133:465–467.
 9. Walther M, O'Brien D, Birch HW. Condyloma acuminata and verrucous carcinoma of the bladder: case report and literature review. *J Urol* 1986;135:362–365.
10. Faysal MH. Squamous cell carcinoma of the bladder. J Urol 1981;126:598–599.
11. Newman DM, Brown JR, Jay AC, et al. Squamous cell carcinoma of the bladder. *J Urol* 1968;112:66–67.
12. Wall RL, Clausen KP. Carcinoma of the urinary bladder in patients receiving cyclophosphamide. *N Engl J Med* 1975;293:271–273.
13. Cheng L, Leibovich BC, Cheville JC, et al. Squamous papilloma of the urinary bladder is unrelated to condyloma acuminata. *Cancer* 2000;88:1679–1686.
14. El Sebai I, Sherif M, El Bolkaimy MN, et al. Verrucous squamous carcinoma of the bladder. *Urol* 1974;4:407–410.
15. Wyatt JK, Craig I. Verrucous carcinoma of urinary bladder. *Urology* 1980;16:97–99.
16. Holck S, Jorgensen L. Verrucous carcinoma of urinary bladder. *Urology* 1983;21:435–437.
17. Botella E, Burgués O, Navarro S, et al. Warty carcinoma arising in condyloma acuminatum of urinary bladder. A case report. *Int J Surg Pathol* 2000;8:253–259.

10

Cystitis

INFECTIOUS

Encrusted Cystitis

Encrusted cystitis refers to inorganic salts being deposited in injured urothelial mucosa as a consequence of urea-splitting bacteria, alkalinizing urine (1). This lesion is most common in women. Histologically, deposits of calcium are present in the lamina propria and the mucosal surface of the bladder is covered with fibrin mixed with calcific, necrotic debris associated with inflammatory cells.

Emphysematous Cystitis

This lesion refers to the presence of gas-filled blebs, predominantly within the lamina propria, which can be seen both at cystoscopy and on the gross examination (2,3). This lesion is more typically found in women, often diabetic, and associated with bacterial infections. Predisposing conditions include trauma, fistula, instrumentation, and urinary stasis. Microscopically, the blebs consist of empty cavities lined by flattened cells surrounded by thin septa; frequently there is an associated foreign body giant cell reaction focally lining the empty spaces.

Fungal Cystitis

Fungal cystitis is uncommon and most often caused by *Candida albicans* (4). Cases of cystitis caused by *Aspergillus* species and other fungi have also been rarely reported. Women are predominantly affected. Most patients are debilitated or are on antibiotic therapy, with diabetic patients being another commonly affected group.

Tuberculosis (Including Bacillus Calmette–Guérin)

Most bladder lesions involved by *Mycobacterium* tuberculosis are secondary to renal involvement (5). Typically the infection begins around ureteral orifices

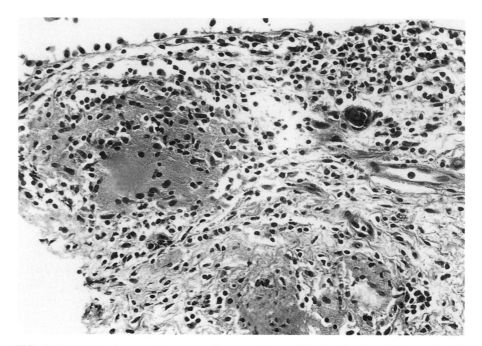

FIG. 10.1. Small submucosal noncaseating granulomas following bacillus Calmette–Guérin immunotherapy.

with superficial ulceration with acute and chronic inflammation and initially noncaseating granulomas. Larger caseating granulomas may follow (efig 923). Late complications include ulcers with fibrosis that can result in ureteral strictures. The histology of tuberculosis more typically seen in current practice is that associated with intravesical bacillus Calmette–Guérin (BCG) immunotherapy for superficial bladder cancer and consists of small, noncaseating granulomas (Fig. 10.1) (efig 924) (see Treatment Related). In patients with a known history of BCG immunotherapy and granulomas on bladder biopsy, we do not perform special stains for organisms.

Schistosomiasis

Schistosomiasis is a chronic disease involving the bladder caused by larvae of *Schistosoma haematobium* (16,17) (Figs. 10.2, 10.3) (Color Plate 11) (efigs 925–933). Coupled adult male and female worms migrate to the veins of the vesical and pelvic plexuses, where they mate and females begin to lay eggs. Involvement of various urogenital organs correlates with the extent of the venous circulation, such that the urinary bladder with a rich venous supply is most heavily infected. Schistosomiasis most commonly occurs in the Middle East and in

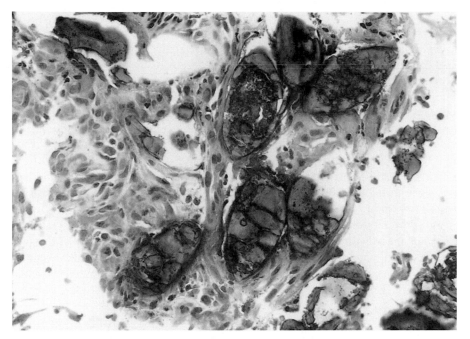

FIG. 10.2. Numerous calcified eggs of schistosomiasis.

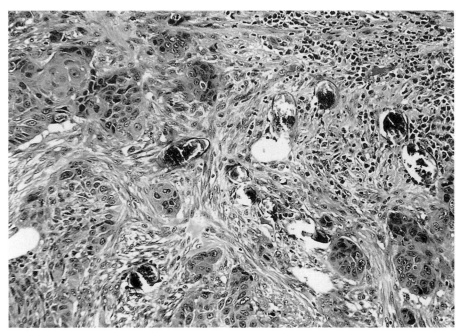

FIG. 10.3. Squamous cell carcinoma (left) associated with calcified eggs of schistosomiasis.

most of the African continent. The highest incidence is where irrigation agriculture is prevalent, such as in the Nile Valley and Delta. The initial response to *S. haematobium* infection is a reaction of the host against the deposition of eggs. This lesion manifests as a granulomatous reaction to the eggs surrounded by numerous eosinophils. *S. haematobium* eggs have terminal spines that differentiate them from other schistosomes, but this is difficult to appreciate in histologic sections. Another differentiating feature is that *S. haematobium* eggshells are not acid-fast, whereas *Schistosoma mansoni* and *Schistosoma japonicum* eggs are. There are several histologic stages of schistosomiasis within the bladder. Recent oviposition gives rise to perioval granulomatous inflammation, which can result in hyperemic polypoid masses. With greater chronicity and less ova position, eggs are destroyed or calcified and inflammation subsides. This gives rise to more fibrous tissue and "sandy patches," in which there is atrophy of the surface epithelium over the schistosomal lesion; old calcified schistosomal eggs buried immediately beneath the mucosa resemble sand seen through shallow water. One may also see schistosomal tubercles that are a manifestation of early active disease, appearing as seedlike, yellowish specks just beneath the urothelium. Each speck reflects a granuloma surrounded by a circle of hyperemia.

Patients with schistosomiasis of the lower urinary tract typically present with painful micturition, frequency, pyuria, and hematuria. Anemia and eosinophilia are common. With greater chronicity, individuals acquire "contracted bladder" syndrome, in which there is intense ova position involving all levels of the muscularis propria with dense fibrosis. Patients present with intractable frequency, painful urination, urgency, and incontinence. Surgery may be indicated when the bladder capacity is significantly reduced, requiring augmentation cystoplasty, using either ileum or colon. Another complication of schistosomiasis within the bladder is ulceration that is attributed to local ischemia caused by schistosomal obliteration of deeper vessels or onset of secondary bacterial infection. Although ulcers may respond to antischistosomal therapy, often total excision by partial cystectomy or endoscopic resection is required. Other nonneoplastic complications include bladder neck obstruction and ureteral strictures. Males are affected more than females in a 4:1 ratio. Carcinogenesis resulting from schistosomal infections is the result of chronic injury, often accompanying bacterial infection, foreign bodies, and urinary concentration of nitrosamines (see Chapter 9).

Malakoplakia

Malakoplakia may affect multiple organs, although the bladder is most commonly involved (6–8). The lesion is characterized by large histiocytes, known as *von Hansemann cells*, and small basophilic extracytoplasmic or intracytoplasmic calculopherules, called *Michaelis–Gutmann bodies* (Fig. 10.4) (efigs 934–940). The bodies are found within the interstitium as well as within histiocytes. Bacteria or bacterial fragments form a nidus for the calcium phosphate

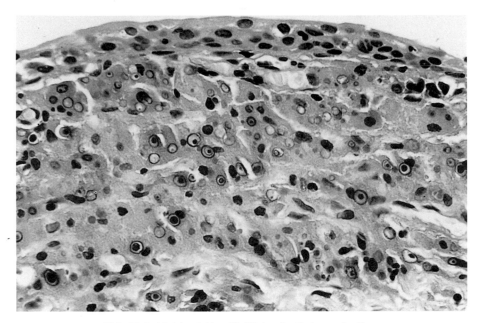

FIG. 10.4. Malakoplakia with Michaelis–Gutmann bodies.

crystals that laminate the Michaelis–Gutmann bodies. A defect in intraphagosomal digestion, which accounts for the unusual immune response, gives rise to malakoplakia (9–15). Electron microscopy reveals intact coliform bacteria and bacterial fragments within phagolysosomes within the foamy histiocytes. The overlying urothelium may be ulcerated, hyperplastic, or metaplastic. In long-standing lesions, the characteristic infiltrate is replaced by fibrosis and scarring. Most patients are middle aged with a female predominance of 4:1. Patients may be debilitated, immunosuppressed, or have other chronic diseases. Cystoscopy reveals mucosal plaques and nodules that, on occasion, become larger masses. There can be significant morbidity, including ureteral strictural stenosis, giving rise to renal obstruction or nonfunction. Management of malakoplakia is primarily based on controlling the urinary tract infections, which stabilizes the disease. Surgery may be necessary as the disease progresses, despite antimicrobial treatment. Malakoplakia may also result in death if it involves both kidneys. Iron and calcium stains can highlight Michaelis–Gutmann bodies, although they are usually quite evident on routine hematoxylin and eosin stained sections.

Viral Cystitis

Both adenovirus and herpes simplex type 2 virus have been associated with hemorrhagic cystitis in a few patients (18,19). Herpes zoster and cytomegalovirus have also been rarely implicated in bladder infections (20,21).

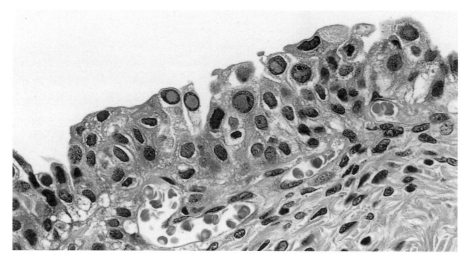

FIG. 10.5. Polyoma virus infection.

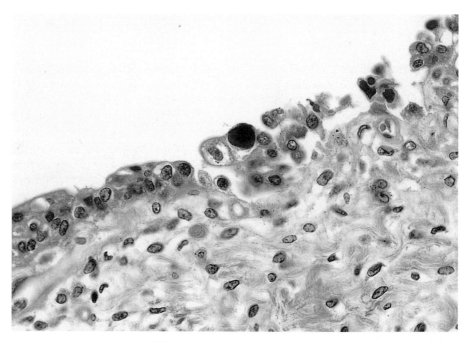

FIG. 10.6. Polyoma virus infection.

Patients with polyoma viruses and bladder involvement are usually immuno-suppressed renal or bone marrow allograft recipients with hemorrhagic cystitis (22,23). Despite the frequency of viruria and intranuclear inclusions seen in urinary cytology specimens in these patients, the identification of inclusions in histologic tissue sections is rare (Figs. 10.5, 10.6) (efigs 941–945).

NONINFECTIOUS

Polypoid Cystitis

Polypoid cystitis may arise as a reaction to any inflammatory insult to the urinary mucosa; a frequently cited etiology is the presence of indwelling catheters (24) (Figs. 10.7–10.14) (efigs 946–997). It occurs equally in males and females, with an age range of 20 months to 79 years. Cystoscopically, it appears either as an area of friable mucosal irregularity or edematous broad papillae. Lesions usually are located adjacent to an inflammatory area. Lesions may be multifocal and can range up to 5 mm in size. Because the urologist can more often recognize the inflammatory nature of the lesion than the pathologist, the pathologist should hesitate diagnosing urothelial carcinoma when the cystoscopic impression is that of an inflammatory lesion.

In its most pronounced form, polypoid cystitis shows extensive submucosal edema with broad bulbous projections termed *bullous cystitis*. Other cases of

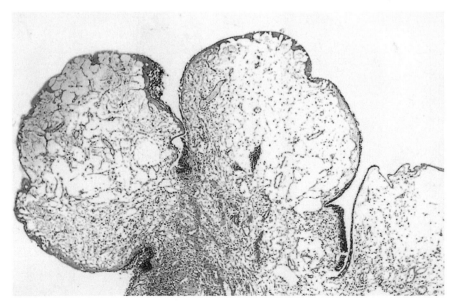

FIG. 10.7. Polypoid cystitis (bullous cystitis).

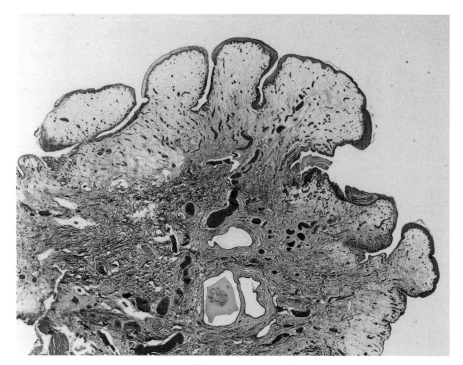

FIG. 10.8. Polypoid cystitis.

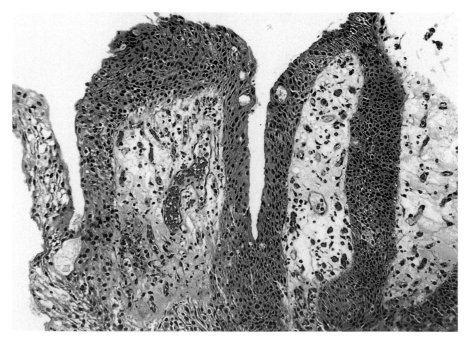

FIG. 10.9. Polypoid cystitis with reactive cytological atypia.

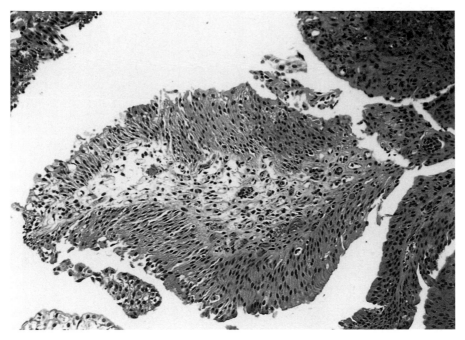

FIG. 10.10. Polypoid cystitis (same case as Figure 10.9). Out of context, isolated frond could be misinterpreted as papillary urothelial neoplasm.

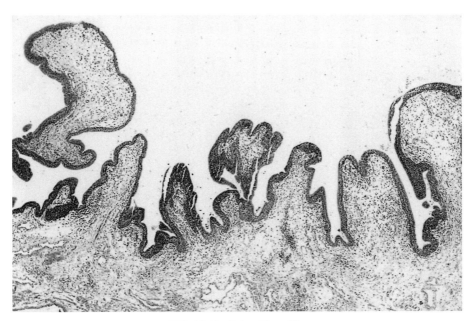

FIG. 10.11. Polypoid cystitis.

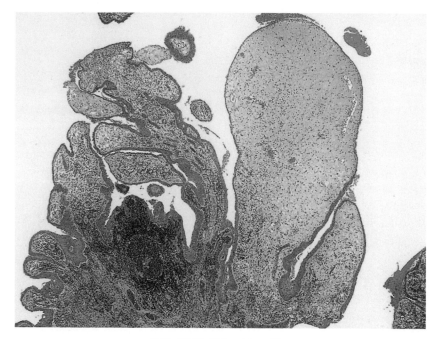

FIG. 10.12. Polypoid cystitis.

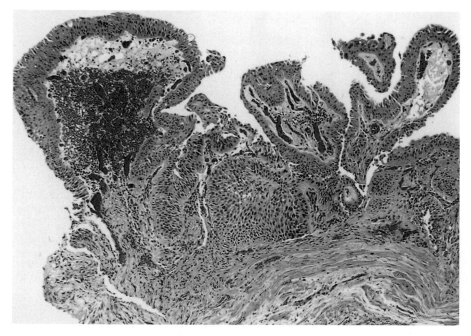

FIG. 10.13. Polypoid cystitis.

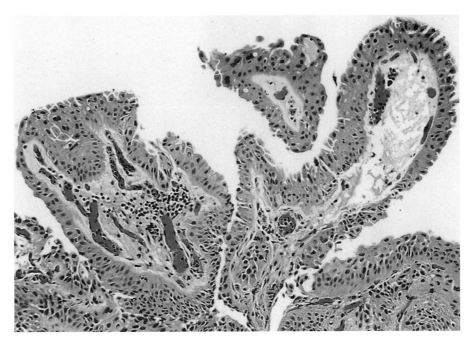

FIG. 10.14. Polypoid cystitis (higher magnification of Figure 10.13). Out of context, isolated frond could be misinterpreted as papillary urothelial neoplasm.

polypoid cystitis may be more difficult to distinguish from urothelial papillary carcinoma. However, these examples of polypoid cystitis still show edematous fibrovascular cores that are broad based in contrast to narrow-necked, thin, and delicate fibrovascular cores of papillary urothelial carcinoma. The fronds in polypoid cystitis do not branch into smaller papillae as can be seen in papillary urothelial carcinoma. With time, fronds of polypoid cystitis lesions become less edematous and are replaced by dense fibrosis often associated with chronic inflammation. These lesions may be referred to as *papillary cystitis* (Figs. 10.15, 10.16). The fibrous tissue in papillary cystitis differs from the delicate loose connective tissue within the fronds of papillary urothelial neoplasms. Out of context, several papillary fronds within polypoid cystitis may closely resemble papillary urothelial carcinoma. However, one must assess the lesion in its entirety and, if overall the lesion is that of polypoid cystitis, one should not overdiagnose isolated papillary fronds as carcinoma.

The urothelial mucosa overlying the edematous stalks may be normal or show reactive urothelial atypia or squamous metaplasia. Polypoid cystitis is a benign lesion without any risk of evolving into carcinoma.

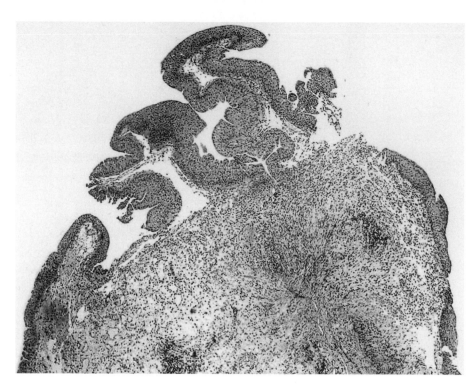

FIG. 10.15. Polypoid cystitis (papillary cystitis).

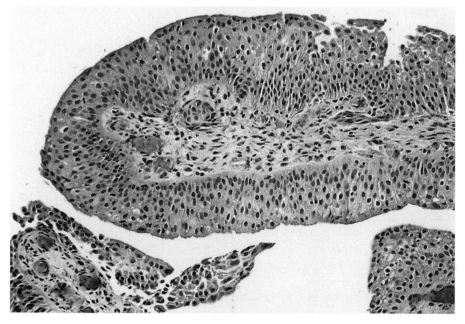

FIG. 10.16. Polypoid cystitis (papillary cystitis) with inflamed fibrous tissue in stalk.

Eosinophilic Cystitis

Eosinophilic cystitis may be seen at all ages and is characterized by dense infiltrate of eosinophils within the lamina propria, submucosa, and, often, muscularis propria (25) (efigs 998, 999). There are two broad settings in which eosinophilic cystitis is found. The most common is that of a subacute, nonspecific inflammatory reaction caused by some other injury. Numerous eosinophils may be seen accompanying carcinomas, areas of prior surgery, and as a response to catheterization. In most of these settings, the eosinophilic infiltrate is not symptomatic and is self-limited. More rarely, eosinophilic cystitis may be seen as a true allergic reaction, such as a reaction to a particular food or drug. Some of these patients may have associated peripheral eosinophilia or associated collagen vascular disease. Treatment in this setting consists of removing the suspected allergen and, in some cases, corticosteroids, anticholinergic drugs, and antiallergic drugs.

Follicular Cystitis

Follicular cystitis, which is more prevalent in children, consists of lymphoid follicles within the lamina propria (26) (Fig. 10.17) (efigs 1000–1005). This

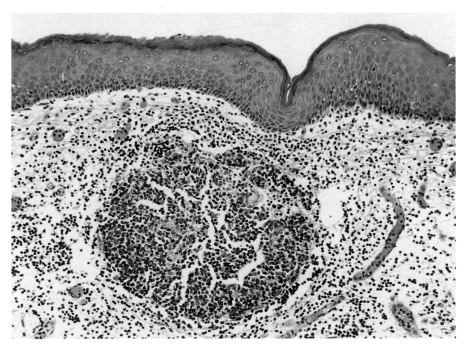

FIG. 10.17. Follicular cystitis with overlying squamous metaplasia.

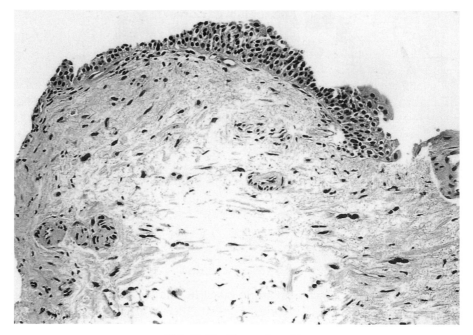

FIG. 10.18. Giant cell cystitis.

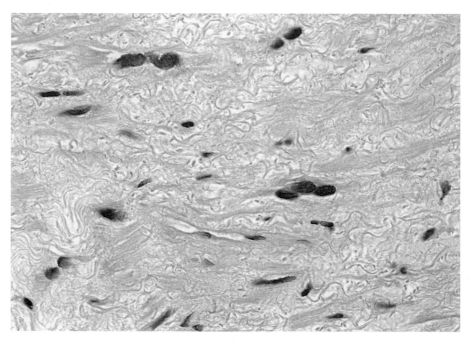

FIG. 10.19. Giant cell cystitis (higher magnification of Figure 10.18).

lesion may be seen grossly as pinpoint white lesions. It is believed to be caused by the presence of bacteria in the bladder and can resolve following antibiotic therapy. Another association is with BCG immunotherapy.

Giant Cell Cystitis

It is not uncommon to find with the lamina propria reactive-appearing stromal cells that are indistinguishable from the fibroblasts associated with radiation (Figs. 10.18, 10.19) (efigs 1006–1009) (27). In contrast to sarcomas, the cells are sparse, have degenerative appearing nuclear atypia, and no mitotic activity.

TREATMENT RELATED

Granulomatous Cystitis Secondary to Bacillus Calmette–Guérin Therapy or Transurethral Biopsy

Urothelial carcinoma in situ (CIS) and high-grade papillary carcinomas are commonly treated with intravesical installations of BCG, which usually induces an intense inflammatory reaction (BCG cystitis) (28–30). It is characterized by the presence of discrete noncaseating granulomas containing epithelioid histiocytes and multinucleated giant cells (efig 924). Rarely do special stains reveal the presence of acid-fast organisms. The granulomas are usually situated in the superficial third of the lamina propria and are associated with an intense lymphocytic infiltrate. The overlying urothelium may show nonspecific reactive atypia or may be partially or entirely denuded. Urine cytology commonly reveals inflammatory cells, including epithelioid histiocytes and occasional giant cells. Many patients undergoing this type of therapy become symptomatic, developing dysuria and occasionally hematuria. In severe cases, patients may develop regional or even systemic lymphadenopathy as well as fever and chills. In these cases biopsy of the enlarged lymph nodes may demonstrate a granulomatous lymphadenitis.

Radiation Cystitis

Radiation cystitis may be acute or chronic and can occur any time the bladder is included in the treatment field. The clinical severity and histologic features of radiation cystitis are both time and dose dependent; 5% of patients receiving 60 Gy to the bladder develop late clinical symptoms of radiation cystitis, whereas 50% of patients suffer the same fate if the dose is 70 Gy (31). Clinically, the acute symptoms of radiation cystitis may appear as early as 4 to 6 weeks after initiation of therapy, whereas late symptoms appear as late as 10 years later (32). The toxic effects of irradiation are enhanced if administered in conjunction with cyclophosphamide (33).

Microscopically the early changes are characterized by marked edema and hyperemia. The edema produces thickened mucosal folds, resulting in a charac-

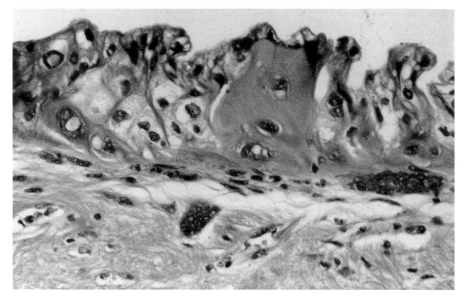

FIG. 10.20. Radiation atypia within urothelium. Atypical cells have degenerative appearing nuclei with vacuolization accompanied by abundant cytoplasm.

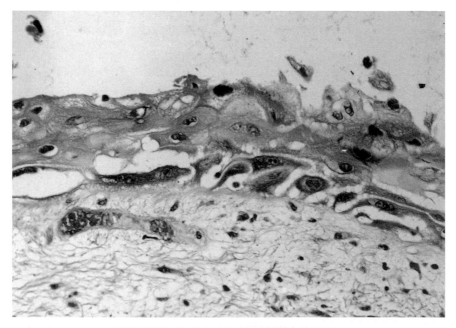

FIG. 10.21. Radiation atypia within urothelium.

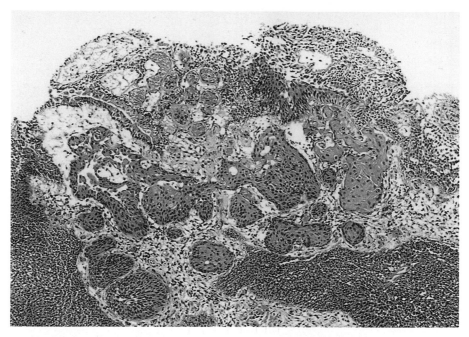

FIG. 10.23. Pseudocarcinomatous hyperplasia resulting from radiotherapy.

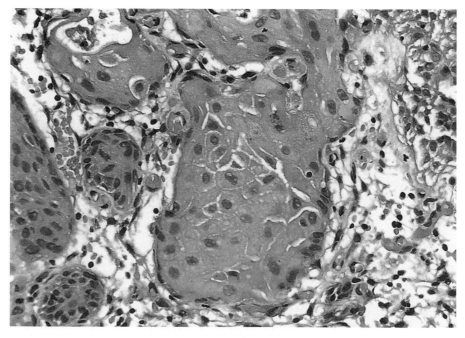

FIG. 10.24. Pseudocarcinomatous hyperplasia resulting from radiotherapy (higher magnification of Figure 10.23).

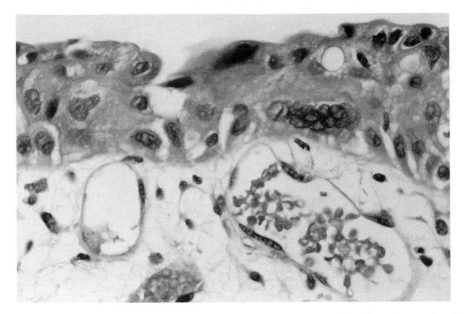

FIG. 10.22. Radiation atypia within urothelium characterized by multinucleated, vacuolated, degenerative appearing nuclei.

teristic gross appearance that was termed *radiation cystitis* by Koss (34). These changes may be accompanied by desquamation and superficial ulceration of the bladder epithelium (35). At this stage, the urothelium can take on atypical cytologic features mimicking and sometimes indistinguishable from CIS although mitotic activity is rare. The cells may become enlarged with prominent, hyperchromatic nuclei (efigs 1010–1015). However, the altered epithelial cells are typically more bizarre than cells of CIS, with giant cells and multinucleated cells that lack the crisp nuclear detail of nonirradiated cells (Figs. 10.20–10.22). In some cases, there is pseudocarcinomatous hyperplasia with epithelial cords and nests that extend into the lamina propria (Figs. 10.23–10.25) (Color Plate 12) (efigs 1016–1030). They are seen adjacent to dilated vascular structures, which frequently contain fibrin. The adjacent stroma also typically is edematous with extravasated erythrocytes, inflammation, and hemosiderin deposition. Given the presence of cytologic atypia, it would be easy to confuse these findings with invasive carcinoma (36). It is said that these changes may disappear over time (33), although we have observed them years after completion of therapy.

Late radiation-induced changes include collagenization of the lamina propria and muscular fibers, myointimal proliferation or hyalinization of the media of arterioles, and, often, ulceration with abundant fibrinous exudate (Fig. 10.26). Atypical fibroblasts are invariably present in the scarred lamina propria. The urothelium may be atrophic or hyperplastic, may undergo squamous metaplasia, and may still exhibit focal radiation-induced atypia (32).

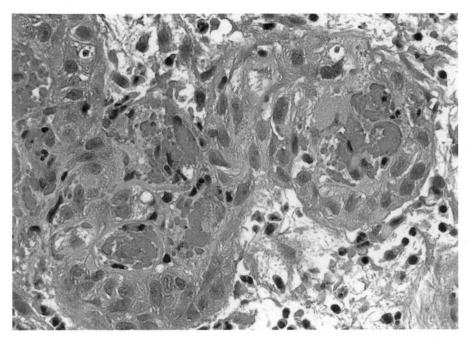

FIG. 10.25. Pseudocarcinomatous hyperplasia resulting from radiotherapy (higher magnification of Figure 10.23). Note epithelial islands wrapping around congested blood vessels and fibrin deposits.

Hemorrhagic Cystitis: Chemotherapy

In the late 1950s, systemic administration of cyclophosphamide was found to cause hemorrhagic cystitis (efigs 1031–1034). At times, hematuria could be massive and uncontrollable, sometimes requiring cystectomy. Philips and colleagues showed that the tissue damage that led to hemorrhagic cystitis was due to a topical effect of the metabolic by-products of cyclophosphamide, which were excreted through the kidney (37). The occurrence of hemorrhagic cystitis appears to be unrelated to dose and was reported in roughly 8% of patients receiving the drug (38,39). Currently, patients are treated with forced fluids and the incidence of hemorrhagic cystitis has been sharply reduced. More recently, another alkylating agent, busulfan, has been implicated as a rare cause of hemorrhagic cystitis (40). Adenovirus infection in children may also result in hemorrhagic cystitis.

Microscopically the bladder is characterized by marked edema and hemorrhage throughout the lamina propria, with extensive ulceration and an associated fibrinopurulent exudate. Where not ulcerated, the epithelium may be thinned and atypical. During the regenerative stage, macrophages and fibroblasts populate

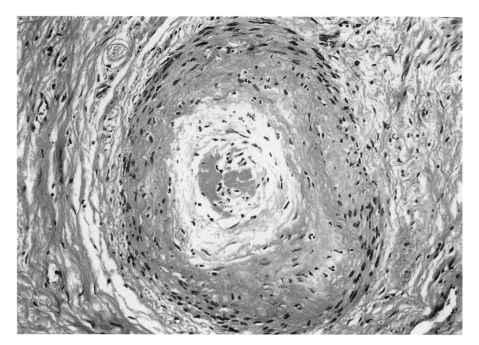

FIG. 10.26. Radiation changes within vessels.

the lamina propria while the overlying epithelium exhibits an increased mitotic rate, increased thickness, and marked atypia (37,39). Intravesical installation of chemotherapeutic agents such as thiotepa and mitomycin C is also able to induce cytologic atypia, which can be confused with CIS, including cytomegaly, pleomorphism, and hyperchromasia (41). Despite these changes, mitotic activity is not evident and superficial (umbrella) cells are preferentially affected. Topical chemotherapy for papillary urothelial carcinoma may also result in truncated papillae (Fig. 2.27). Clinical trials evaluating the efficacy of yet another agent as an intravesical chemotherapeutic agent, gemcitabine, are ongoing; we have found that it induces similar morphologic changes that mimic carcinoma.

Posttransurethral Resection

A nonspecific granulomatous inflammation with foreign body giant cells can also be seen following transurethral resections (42,43) (Fig. 10.27) (efigs 1035–1037). In severe cases, this procedure may lead to the development of necrotizing palisading granulomas (efigs 1038–1042). The necrotic center is surrounded by epithelioid histiocytes with occasional foreign body–type giant cells. Depending on the extent of the resection, the surrounding bladder wall is fibrotic with obliteration of the normal anatomic landmarks.

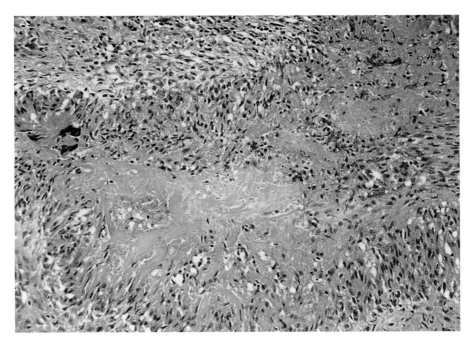

FIG. 10.27. Posttransurethral resection granuloma.

INTERSTITIAL CYSTITIS

Interstitial cystitis is a chronic inflammatory process affecting the urinary bladder, characterized by a constellation of symptoms including urinary frequency, nocturia, urgency, suprapubic pressure, and pelvic and bladder pain. The diagnosis of interstitial cystitis is complex, one that is frequently made after several visits by the patient to several different physicians. Because the diagnosis is based mainly on the clinical findings and remains more or less one that is achieved after excluding several other possibilities, the question of whether there is a role for the surgical pathologist is frequently asked. The most critical tasks for the pathologist are to (a) accurately rule out other forms of cystitis and CIS, lesions that clinically and cystoscopically may mimic interstitial cystitis, and (b) in a documented case, provide correlations of histology with cystoscopic findings and clinical features. The ultimate diagnosis of interstitial cystitis is made after clinical and pathologic correlation, but histologic clues may help alert the unsuspecting urologist.

Interstitial cystitis is typically characterized by a varying symptom complex, which includes suprapubic pain, urinary frequency, nocturia, urinary urgency, and pain on bladder filling, which is typically relieved on voiding. Greater than 90% of patients are women and the disease most commonly affects middle-aged and old women. The etiology of interstitial cystitis is currently unknown despite extensive research efforts (44–46). The urine, when cultured, is sterile for organisms detectable by routine laboratory workup. Interestingly, many patients have autoimmune diseases (e.g., lupus erythematosus) and, hence, autoimmune diseases have also been considered to be contributory to the pathogenesis. Trauma, structural defects, infections, and immunologic derangements, or combinations thereof, are thought to play a role in etiology and pathogenesis (46–48).

If interstitial cystitis is being considered, the diagnostic evaluation includes a urinalysis, urine microscopy, cytology, culture, and cystoscopy with biopsy. The presence of submucosal hemorrhages, that is, "glomerulations," after bladder distention or the presence of Hunner ulcer may be considered to be diagnostic of interstitial cystitis in a patient having the symptom complex. Urodynamic studies may be performed to document decreased bladder filling capacity.

Cystoscopically, the disease is categorized as the *nonulcer or early disease* and the classic Hunner ulcer. The nonulcer disease exhibits multiple microhemorrhages within the lamina propria that are referred to as *glomerulations*. In the classic phase, the bladder on cystoscopy displays single or multiple patches of reddened mucosa with small blood vessels radiating from a central scar. Under hydrodistention, the mucosa ruptures, resulting in oozing of blood from the mucosal margins on the bottom of the ulcer; this is referred to as *Hunner ulcer*.

There are no characteristic histologic features for interstitial cystitis (49–51). In routine cystoscopic biopsies, suburothelial edema and telangiectasia are con-

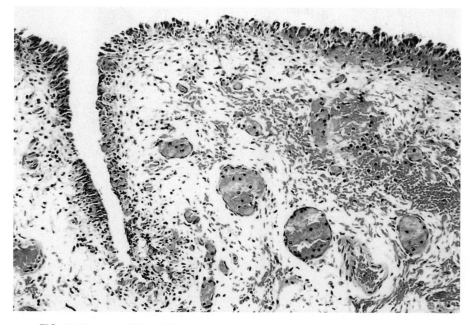

FIG. 10.28. Interstitial cystitis, nonulcerative type with lamina propria hemorrhages.

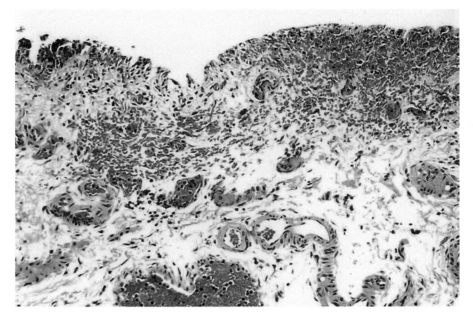

FIG. 10.29. Interstitial cystitis, nonulcerative type with lamina propria hemorrhages.

stantly observed regardless whether the disease is "classic" or of the "nonulcer" form. The edema is striking and out of proportion to the existing inflammation. The findings in nonulcer patients are usually meager and limited to mucosal ruptures or tears and suburothelial hemorrhages that correspond to the cystoscopically observed glomerulations (Figs. 10.28, 10.29) (efigs 1043–1049). The mucosal ruptures may be single or multiple and vary from only superficially involving the lamina propria to those extending deeply up to the muscularis propria. Most patients show suburothelial hemorrhage; however, the hemorrhage may or may not necessarily be associated with overlying mucosal rupture. Nonspecific proliferative changes including von Brunn nests and cystitis cystica may be present.

In patients with Hunner ulcer, the morphologic changes are more marked (Figs. 10.30–10.32) (efigs 1050–1060). The mucosal ulcers are often covered by debris, fibrin, inflammatory cells, and red blood cells. The ulcers vary in thickness, but usually involve the upper half of the lamina propria. The ulcer base is comprised of granulation tissue. The rest of the lamina propria shows a fairly moderate to marked inflammatory infiltrate with lymphoid aggregates occasionally forming germinal centers. The inflammation is usually diffuse, but perineural inflammatory cells may be seen in 70% of the patients (chronic perineuritis) (49). Hemorrhage within the lamina propria is usually marked in patients with ulcer disease and is seen frequently in association with the ulcer, but it may

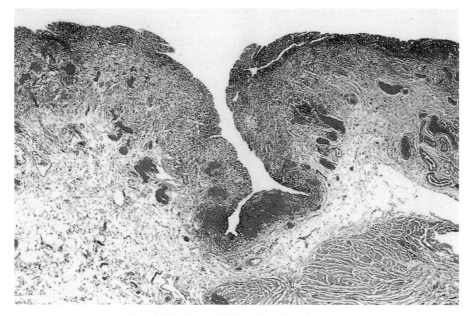

FIG. 10.30. Interstitial cystitis, ulcerative type.

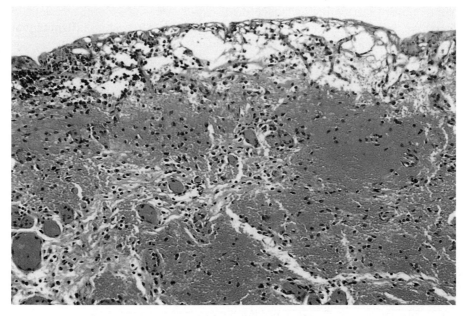

FIG. 10.31. Interstitial cystitis, ulcerative type with surface granulation tissue.

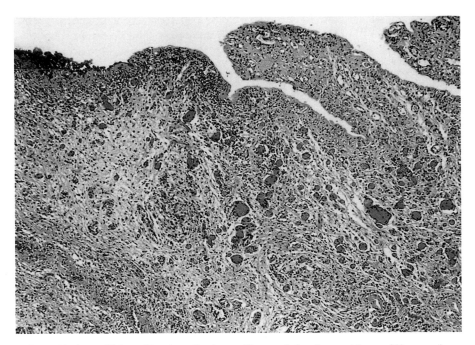

FIG. 10.32. Interstitial cystitis, ulcerative type with granulation tissue at base of Hunner ulcer.

also be seen in areas without significant inflammation. The lamina propria may also show fibrosis and vasculitis.

The inflammation is generally chronic and nonspecific in nature with a variable density and distribution of lymphocytes, macrophages, and plasma cells. Acute inflammation and eosinophils may be seen on rare occasions, but this is invariably seen in patients with ulcers. Besides chronic perineuritis, nerve hypertrophy and proliferation of nerves may be observed. In long-standing cases, fibrosis and inflammation may be seen in the muscularis propria, a finding that correlates with the decreased bladder capacity seen in advanced stages of the disease. The perivesical fat usually lacks significant inflammation. A high mast cell count in the muscularis propria of the bladder (detrusor muscle) was initially touted as a diagnostic histopathologic feature for interstitial cystitis and, hence, the term *detrusor mastocytosis* was advocated. The significance of mast cells is controversial, in that mast cell counts in patients with interstitial cystitis overlap with counts in patients with bladder inflammation of other causes (52,53). Also, most mast cell counts do not correlate with clinical symptoms, cystoscopic findings, or response to therapy. Mast cell counts exceeding 28 mast cells/mm^2 in the detrusor muscle are thought to strongly support a diagnosis of interstitial cystitis; the counts within the lamina propria are less specific. Giemsa, toluidine blue, Leder stain, Bismarck brown, Alcian blue at pH1, and monoclonal antibody CD-

117 are frequently used to identify mast cells. Because there is no clear-cut role of mast cell count in the diagnosis of interstitial cystitis and because of the relatively cumbersome process for its evaluation, we do not routinely perform mast cell counts.

A wide range of differential diagnostic possibilities must be considered while ruling out interstitial cystitis. Although the list is extensive, not all of them are active considerations in most cases. CIS is an important differential diagnostic consideration. Although 25% of patients with CIS may be asymptomatic, most patients, especially those with de novo CIS, present with frequency, dysuria, nocturia, and suprapubic fullness. Cystoscopically, the involved areas exhibit erythema or granularity, which also mimic interstitial cystitis. The extensive mucosal denudation that frequently occurs with CIS may result in a biopsy appearance of ulceration, vascular congestion, and inflammation resembling interstitial cystitis. When the urothelium is absent or scant, multiple levels should be obtained to look for atypical cells and to rule out the possibility of CIS. Other forms of cystitis in the differential diagnosis include hemorrhagic cystitis, which is often catastrophic in presentation, eosinophilic cystitis, and radiation cystitis.

REFERENCES

1. Meria P, Desgrippes A, Arfi C, et al. Encrusted cystitis and pyelitis. *J Urol* 1998;160:3–9.
2. Patel NP, Lavengood RW, Fernandes M, et al. Gas-forming infections in genitourinary tract. *Urology* 1992;39:341–345.
3. Quint HJ, Drach GW, Rappaport WD, et al. Emphysematous cystitis: a review of the spectrum of disease. *J Urol* 1992;147:134–137.
4. Wise GJ, Silver DA. Fungal infections of the genitourinary system. *J Urol* 1993;149:1377–1388.
5. Christensen WI. Genitourinary tuberculosis: review of 102 cases, *Medicine* 1974;53:377–390.
6. Melicow MM. Malakoplakia. Report of case, review of literature. *J Urol* 1957;78:33–40.
7. Smith BH. Malakoplakia of the urinary tract. A study of 24 cases. *Am J Clin Pathol* 1965;43:409–417.
8. McClure J. Malakoplakia. *J Pathol* 1983;140:275–330.
9. Lou TY, Teplitz C. Malakoplakia: pathogenesis and ultrastructural morphogenesis. A problem of altered macrophage (phagolysomal) response. *Hum Pathol* 1974;5:191–207.
10. Damjanov I, Katz SM. Malakoplakia. *Pathol Annu* 1981;16:103–126.
11. Stanton MJ, Maxted W. Malakoplakia: A study of the literature and current concepts of pathogenesis, diagnosis and treatment. *J Urol* 1981;125:139–146.
12. Lewin KJ, Fair WR, Steigbigel RT, et al. Clinical and laboratory studies into the pathogenesis of malakoplakia. *J Clin Pathol* 1976;29:354–363.
13. Abdou NI, NaPombejara C, Sagawa A, et al. Malakoplakia: evidence for monocyte lysosomal abnormality correctable by cholinergic agonist in vitro and in vivo. *N Engl J Med* 1977;297:1413–1419.
14. Qualman SJ, Gupta PK, Mendelsohn G. Intracellular *Escherichia coli* in urinary malakoplakia: a reservoir of infection and its therapeutic implications. *Am J Clin Pathol* 1984;81:35–42.
15. Steven S, McClure J. The histochemical features of the Michaelis–Gutmann body and a consideration of the pathophysiological mechanisms of its formation. *J Pathol* 1982;137:119–127.
16. Ghoneim MA. Bilharziasis of the genitourinary tract. *BJU Int* 2002;89[Suppl 1]:22–30.
17. Zahran MM, Kamel M, Mooro H, et al. Bilharziasis of urinary bladder and ureter: comparative histopathologic study. *Urology* 1976;8:73–79.
18. Mufson MA, Belshe RB. A review of adenoviruses in the etiology of acute hemorrhagic cystitis. *J Urol* 1976;115:191–194.

19. De Hertogh DA, Brettman LR. Hemorrhagic cystitis due to herpes simplex virus as a marker of disseminated herpes infection. *Am J Med* 1988;84:62–65.
20. Richmond W. The genital-urinary manifestations of herpes zoster, 3 case reports under review of the literature. *Br J Urol* 1974;46:193–200.
21. Wong T-W, Warner NE. Cytomegalic inclusion disease in adults. Report of 14 cases with review of literature. *Arch Pathol* 1962;74:403–422.
22. Apperley JF, Rice SJ, Bishop JA, et al. Late-onset hemorrhagic cystitis associated with urinary excretions of polyoma viruses after bone marrow transplantation. *Transplantation* 1987;43:108–112.
23. Vogeli TA, Peinemann F, Burdach S, et al. Urological treatment and clinical course of B-K polyoma virus-associated hemorrhagic cystitis in children after bone marrow transplantation. *Eur Urol* 1999; 36:252–257.
24. Young RH. Papillary and polypoid cystitis: a report of 8 cases. *Am J Surg Pathol* 1988;12:542–546.
25. Verhagen PCMS, Nikkels PGJ, de Jong TPVM. Eosinophilic cystitis. *Arch Dis Child* 2001;84: 344–346.
26. Hansson S, Hanson E, Hjälmås K, et al. Follicular cystitis in girls with untreated asymptomatic or covert bacteriuria. *J Urol* 1990;143:330–332.
27. Wells HG. Giant cells in cystitis. *Arch Pathol Lab Med* 1938;26:32–43.
28. Lage JM, Bauer WC, Kelley DR. Histological parameters and pitfalls in the interpretation of bladder biopsies in bacillus Calmette–Guérin treatment of superficial bladder cancer. *J Urol* 1986;135: 916–919.
29. Pagano F, Bassi P, Milani C. Pathologic and structural changes in the bladder after BCG intravesical therapy in men. *Prog Clin Biol Res* 1989;310:81–91.
30. Betz SA, See WA, Cohen MB. Granulomatous inflammation in bladder wash specimens after bacillus Calmete–Guérin therapy for transitional cell carcinoma of the bladder. *Am J Clin Pathol* 1993;99: 244–248.
31. Rubin R. *Radiation biology and radiation pathology syllabus*. Chicago: American College of Radiology, 1975:210.
32. Fajardo LF, Berthrong M. Radiation injury in surgical pathology. Part 1. *Am J Surg Pathol* 1978;2: 159–195.
33. Jayalakshmamma B, Pinkel D. Urinary bladder toxicity following pelvic irradiation and simultaneous cyclophosphamide therapy. *Cancer* 1976;38:701–707.
34. Koss LG. Tumors of the urinary bladder fascicle 11 (2nd series). In: *Altas of tumor pathology*. Washington, DC: Armed Forces Institute of Pathology, 1975:99–102.
35. Warren S. Effects of radiation on normal tissues. Effects of radiation on the urinary system. *Arch Pathol* 1942;34:1079–1084.
36. Balker PM, Young RH. Radiation-induced pseudocarcinomatous proliferations of the urinary bladder: a report of 4 cases. *Hum Pathol* 2000;31:678–683.
37. Philips FS, Sternberg SS, Cronin AP, et al. Cyclophosphamide and urinary bladder toxicity. *Cancer Res* 1961;21:1577–1589.
38. Lawrence HJ, Simone J, Aur RJA. Cyclophosphamide-induced hemorrhagic cystitis in children with leukemia. *Cancer* 1975;36:1572–1576.
39. Beyer-Boon ME, De Voogt HJ, et al. The effects of cyclophosphamide treatment on the epithelium and stroma of the urinary bladder. *Eur J Cancer* 1978;14:1029–1035.
40. Pode D, Perlberg S, Steiner D. Busulfan-induced hemorrhagic cystitis. *J Urol* 1983;130:347–348.
41. Murphy WM, Soloway MS, Lin CJ. Morphologic effects of thio-tepa on mammalian urothelium, changes in abnormal cells. *Acta Cytol* 1978;22:550–554.
42. Spagnolo DV, Waring PM. Bladder granulomata after bladder surgery. *Am J Surg Pathol* 1986;86: 430–437.
43. Eble JN, Banks ER. Post-surgery necrobiotic granulomas of urinary bladder. *Urology* 1990;35: 454–457.
44. Sant GR. Interstitial cystitis. *Curr Opin Obstet Gynecol* 1997;9:332–336.
45. Ochs RL. Autoantibodies and interstitial cystitis. *Clin Lab Med* 1997;17:571–579.
46. Sant GR, Hanno PM. Interstitial cystitis: current issues and controversies in diagnosis. *Urology* 2001;57[Suppl 6A]:82–88.
47. Gillenwater JY, Wein AJ: Summary of the National Institute of Arthritis, Diabetes, Digestive, and Kidney Diseases Workshop on Interstitial Cystitis. National Institute of Health, Bethesda, Maryland, August 28-29, 1987. *J Urol* 1988;140:203–206.

48. Elbadawi A. Interstitial cystitis: a critique of current concepts with a new proposal for pathologic diagnosis and pathogenesis. *Urology* 1997;49:14–40.
49. Johansson SL, Fall M: Clinical features and spectrum of light microscopic changes in interstitial cystitis *J Urol* 1990;143:1118–1124.
50. Tomaszewski JE, Landis JR, Russack V, et al. Biopsy features are associated with primary symptoms in interstitial cystitis: results from the interstitial cystitis database study. *Urology* 2001;57[Suppl 6A]: 67–81.
51. Johannsson SL. Interstitial cystitis. *Mod Pathol* 1993;6:738–742.
52. Larsen S, Thompson SA, Hald T, et al. Mast cells in interstitial cystitis. *Br J Urol* 1982;54:283–286.
53. Theoharides TC, Duraisamy K, Sant GR. Mast cell involvement in interstitial cystitis: a review of human and experimental evidence. *Urology* 2001;57[Suppl 6A]:47–55.

11

Mesenchymal Tumors and Tumor-Like Lesions

Rare cases of benign mesenchymal neoplasms of the urinary tract have been described, although they are less common than their malignant counterparts. Primary sarcomas of the urinary bladder are rare, but more common in males than females. Most are of muscle origin and comprise less than 0.04% of all malignant tumors of the urinary bladder (1–3). Myosarcomas may occur in any age group, but rhabdomyosarcomas predominate in children whereas leiomyosarcomas predominate in adults.

LEIOMYOMA

Leiomyoma is the most common of this group, exhibiting the same morphologic features seen at other sites (4–6) (Figs. 11.1, 11.2) (efigs 1061–1063).

LEIOMYOSARCOMA

Leiomyosarcomas are more commonly seen in adults, although cases have been reported in children (1,3,4,7). The tumors are usually well circumscribed, and may protrude into the lumen and ulcerate the overlying urothelium. Size is variable, although some may measure up to 20 cm. They occur more frequently in males than in females in a ratio of 2:1. Morphologic features are identical to those seen in other sites, including the presence of interlacing fascicles of spindle cells with variable amounts of eosinophilic cytoplasm with mild to marked nuclear atypia (Figs. 11.3–11.5) (efigs 1064–1070). Some tumors may have prominent myxoid change. Most cases demonstrate tumor necrosis and mitotic activity of ten per 10 high-power fields or more. From a practical point of view, we use the same criteria applied in uterine primaries to assess the biologic potential of vesical leiomyosarcomas.

Sarcomatoid carcinoma may mimic leiomyosarcoma and must be excluded by adequate sampling of the specimen and appropriate histochemical, immunohis-

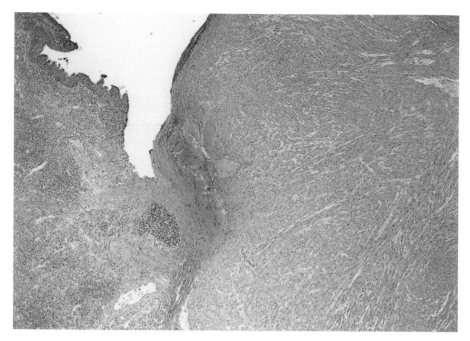

FIG. 11.1. Leiomyoma.

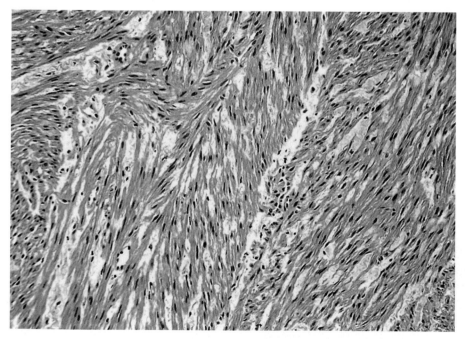

FIG. 11.2. Leiomyoma (higher magnification of Figure 11.1).

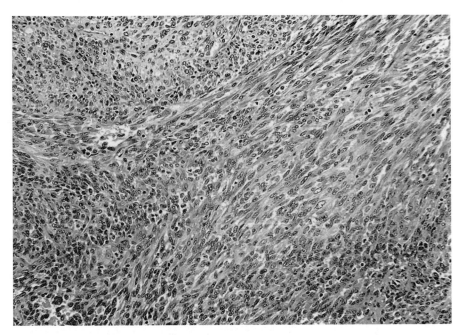

FIG. 11.3. Leiomyosarcoma.

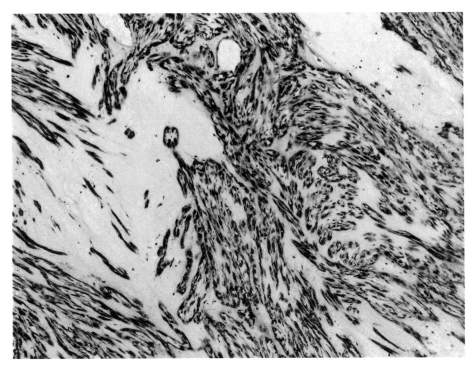

FIG. 11.4. Myxoid leiomyosarcoma.

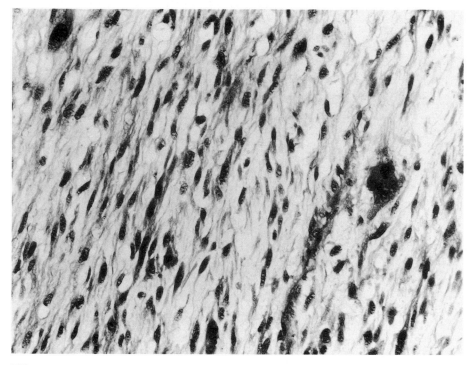

FIG. 11.5. Myxoid leiomyosarcoma. In contrast to inflammatory myofibroblastic tumor, this lesion lacks inflammation and reactive fibroblastic-appearing cells and rather shows scattered hyperchromatic pleomorphic nuclei.

TABLE 11.1. *Spindle cell neoplasms of the bladder: immunoreactivity*

Antibody	RMS	LMS	SFT	IMT	SC[a]
Vim	+	+	+	+	+
SMA (1A4)	–/+	+	–/+	+/–	–
MCA (HHF-35)	+	+	–/+	+	–
Desmin	+	+/–	–	–/+	–
Myogenin	+	–	–	–	–
CD-34	–	–	+	–	–
Bcl-2	–	–/+	+	–/+	–/+
Alk	–	–	–	+/–	–
EMA	–	–	–	–	+/–
CAM 5.2	–	–/+	–	–/+	+/–
34BE12	–	–	–	–	+/–

+, positive in >75% of cases; +/–, positive in >50% of cases; –/+, positive in <50% of cases; –, negative in <5% of cases; EMA, epithelial membrane antigen (clone MC5); IMT, inflammatory myofibroblastic tumor; LMS, leiomyosarcoma; MCA, muscle common actin (clone HHF-35); RMS, rhabdomyosarcoma; SC, Sarcomatoid carcinoma; SFT, solitary fibrous tumor; SMA, smooth muscle actin (clone 1A4); Vim, vimentin.
[a]Sarcomatoid carcinomas with mesenchymal differentiation may express muscle markers.

tochemical, and electron microscopic studies. Leiomyosarcomas of the bladder are so rare that this diagnosis should be made only after excluding all other possibilities, particularly carcinoma. One must also rule out reactive spindle cell lesions that may occur after local surgery or trauma. These reactive lesions are composed of spindle cells that may express smooth muscle markers by immunohistochemistry but are of myofibroblastic origin (see later text). More than two thirds of leiomyosarcomas demonstrate immunoreactivity of both smooth muscle actin (1A4) and muscle-specific actin (HHF-35). Desmin is positive in less than 50% of cases, whereas cytokeratins and epithelial membrane antigen are usually negative. It has been suggested that caldesmon is positive in leiomyosarcomas but negative in myofibroblastic lesions (8) (Table 11.1).

RHABDOMYOSARCOMA

In children, 20% to 27% of rhabdomyosarcomas arise most commonly in the genitourinary tract, bladder, prostate, and paratesticular regions as primary sites in males and in the bladder and vagina in females (9–12) (Fig. 11.6) (Color Plate 13) (efigs 1071–1073). The mean age at diagnosis for vesical rhabdomyosarcomas is 4 years. Most are embryonal rhabdomyosarcomas and exophytic (polypoid), with or without a "botryoid" component. Microscopically the botryoid variant of rhab-

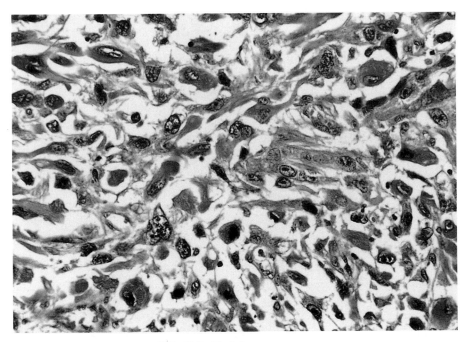

FIG. 11.6. Rhabdomyosarcoma.

domyosarcoma has a superficial condensation of tumor cells, including strap cells and rhabdomyoblasts, located immediately beneath the urothelium. The underlying stroma is hypocellular and myxoid. In other polypoid tumors, the neoplastic cells are diffusely distributed throughout. A significant percentage of vesical rhabdomyosarcomas do not have an exophytic component and in these the tumor cells infiltrate the bladder wall diffusely (12). The spindle cell and alveolar variants of rhabdomyosarcoma may be rarely encountered. Typical rhabdomyoblasts and cross striations are seen frequently in exophytic rhabdomyosarcomas but rarely in the spindle cell and alveolar types. Rare cases of vesical rhabdomyosarcoma have been described in adults and these may have embryonal, pleomorphic, or alveolar patterns (11). Rhabdomyosarcoma should enter in the differential diagnosis of all spindle and myxoid lesions of the genitourinary tract in the pediatric age group. Tumor cells are at least focally immunoreactive for desmin and myogenin, the latter in a nuclear distribution. Immunoreactivity for myoglobin is also diagnostic, although it is positive in a minority of cases (Table 11.1).

In general, rhabdomyosarcomas have a poor prognosis in adults. Combination therapy with surgery and chemotherapy has greatly improved survival in the pediatric age group. Studies have suggested that exophytic rhabdomyosarcomas have a better prognosis than those that infiltrate the bladder wall diffusely (12). Interestingly, treated tumors commonly exhibit morphologic evidence of "maturation" as evidenced by a greater number of myoblasts and cross striations.

INFLAMMATORY MYOFIBROBLASTIC TUMOR AND POSTOPERATIVE SPINDLE CELL NODULE

Several lesions involve the urinary bladder and mimic sarcoma or sarcomatoid carcinoma. They have been described under a variety of names but share many histologic and clinical features (Figs. 11.7–11.15) (Color Plate 14) (efigs 1074–1123). In 1984, Proppe and colleagues reported on nine cases of spindle cell tumors, two of which involved the bladder and three the prostatic urethra, all appearing within months of a transurethral resection (TUR) (13). They named the lesions *postoperative spindle-cell nodules of the genitourinary tract*. These apparently benign proliferative lesions are characterized histologically by plump or elongated spindle cells, which infiltrate the bladder wall and focally can destroy muscle. The lesion can be quite cellular. A prominent feature of these tumors is a delicate network of small blood vessels in an edematous or myxoid stroma with little to moderate collagen deposition. Mitotic figures may be present and even frequent, but they are not atypical. The surface urothelium is usually ulcerated with an acute inflammatory cell infiltrate superficially and chronic inflammatory infiltrate scattered throughout the remainder of the lesion.

FIG. 11.8. Postoperative spindle cell nodule (inflammatory myofibroblastic tumor). Note mitotic figures (*arrows*).

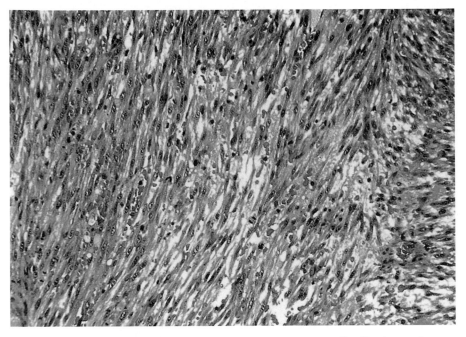

FIG. 11.7. Postoperative spindle cell nodule (inflammatory myofibroblastic tumor).

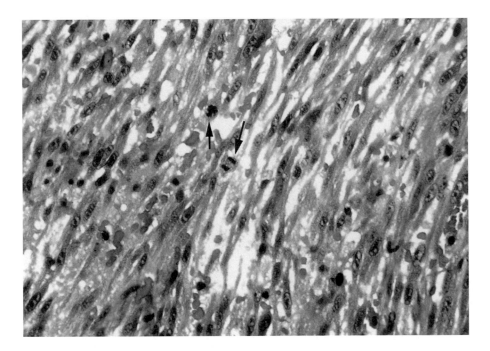

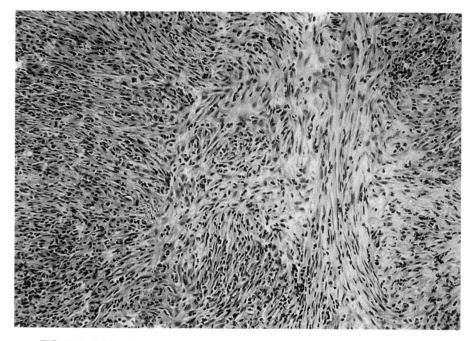

FIG. 11.9. Inflammatory myofibroblastic tumor with interspersed inflammatory cells.

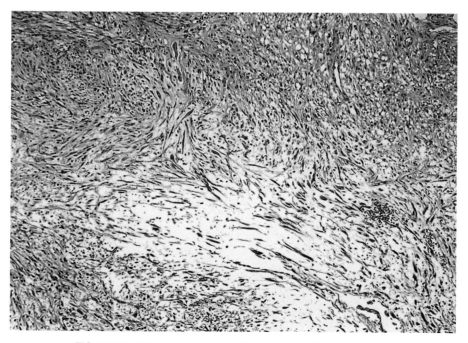

FIG. 11.10. Inflammatory myofibroblastic tumor with myxoid areas.

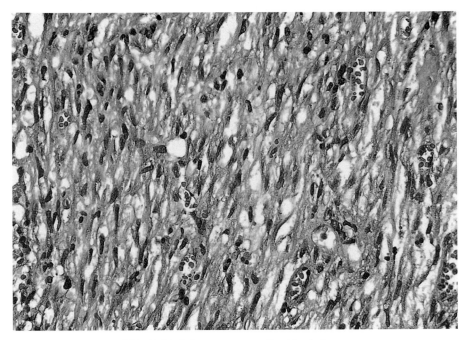

FIG. 11.11. Inflammatory myofibroblastic tumor.

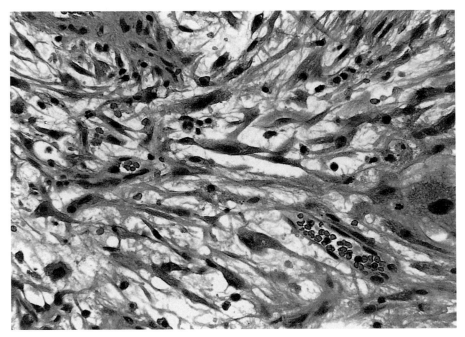

FIG. 11.12. Inflammatory myofibroblastic tumor with tissue culture-like cells.

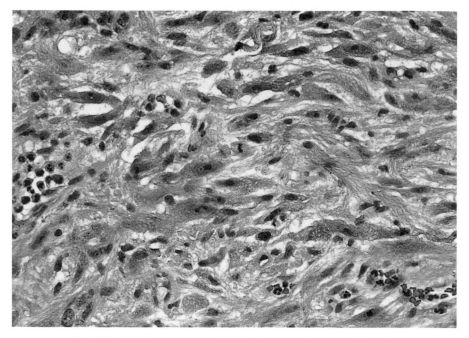

FIG. 11.13. Inflammatory myofibroblastic tumor (note mitotic figure).

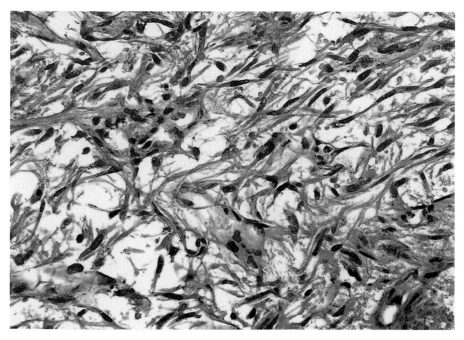

FIG. 11.14. Inflammatory myofibroblastic tumor with tissue culture-like cells.

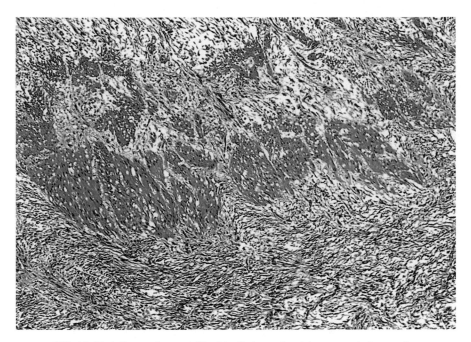

FIG. 11.15. Inflammatory myofibroblastic tumor involving muscularis propria.

Histologically similar lesions were described by other authors and called *inflammatory pseudotumor* (14,15) and *pseudosarcomatous fibromyxoid tumor* (16), and *pseudosarcomatous myofibroblastic proliferation* (17). A similar pseudosarcomatous lesion was reported by Roth (18). The lesions were either pedunculated or polypoid, with a low mitotic rate. They appeared either spontaneously or in a background of chronic cystitis and differed from the cases reported by Proppe in that they were not necessarily related to a recent operative procedure. It is currently believed that these tumors represent a single lesion or at least closely related entities, all being of myofibroblastic origin; most authors use the term *inflammatory myofibroblastic tumor* (IMT) to describe them. A few studies have demonstrated clonality, suggesting that they are neoplastic rather than reactive in nature, a possible exception being those that occur immediately following instrumentation. In support of this finding, we have seen rare examples of morphologically malignant myofibroblastic tumors of the bladder and urethra with atypical mitoses and tumor necrosis, although none of these cases have yet developed metastases.

The differential diagnosis usually is with leiomyosarcoma and sarcomatoid (spindle cell) carcinoma (19–22). Invasive or metastatic urothelial carcinoma may also incite a pseudosarcomatous stromal reaction, which may be confused with a myofibroblastic proliferation or with sarcoma (19). A reactive pseudosarcomatous lesion should always be suspected of postoperative spindle cell lesions involving the bladder. The best clues to their benign nature are a delicate but abundant vascular network, absence of atypical mitotic figures, edematous or myxoid stroma, and a sprinkling of chronic inflammatory cells deep within the lesion. Tumor cells will usually have the features of reactive myofibroblasts with large, epithelioid nuclei and abundant eosinophilic cytoplasm. Immunohistochemical studies or electron microscopy may be of help to prove the myofibroblastic nature of the cells (21–23). Nevertheless, extreme caution is warranted in the interpretation of the immunohistochemical stains because proliferating myofibroblasts may be positive for cytokeratins, vimentin, and actin (20), although not caldesmon or epithelial membrane antigen (Table 11.1). IMTs are said to express anaplastic lymphoma kinase (ALK) by immunohistochemistry (24). This ALK overexpression goes along with the finding of a recurrent translocation involving chromosome band 2p23, site of the ALK gene, in these tumors. However, this polyclonal antibody (ALK-11) does not work consistently.

MISCELLANEOUS BENIGN MESENCHYMAL TUMORS

Rare examples of hemangioma have been reported in the bladder, which must be differentiated from bladder angiosarcoma (25,26) (Figs. 11.16, 11.17) (efigs 1124–1132). Other benign mesenchymal tumors arising at this site include fibroma (27) and neurofibroma (28) (Figs. 11.18–11.20) (efigs 1133–1137).

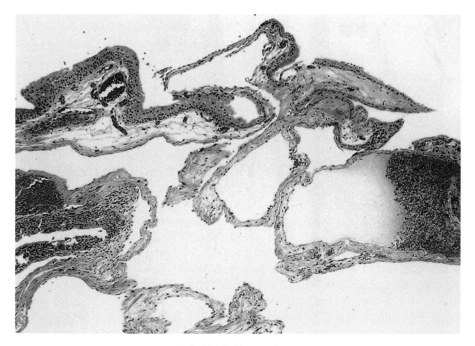

FIG. 11.16. Hemangioma.

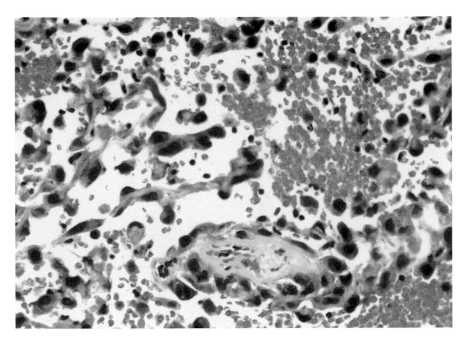

FIG. 11.17. Angiosarcoma.

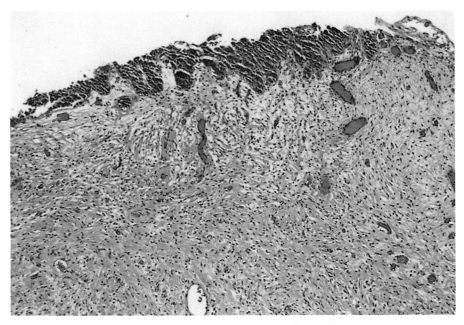

FIG. 11.18. Neurofibroma within lamina propria.

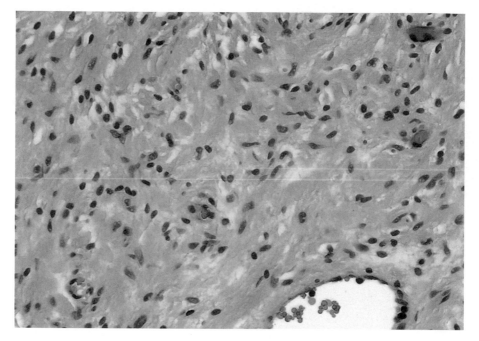

FIG. 11.19. Neurofibroma (higher magnification of Figure 11.18).

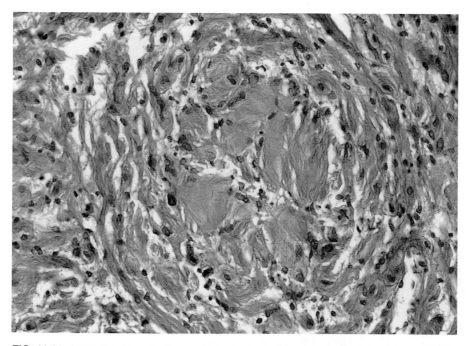

FIG. 11.20. Neurofibroma with Wagner-Meissner body (higher magnification of Figure 11.18).

Several cases of hemangiopericytoma have been described arising within the urinary bladder as well, as have granular cell tumors (29–31). They usually behave in a benign fashion after complete local excision.

SOLITARY FIBROUS TUMOR

Solitary fibrous tumors (SFTs) may originate within the pelvis, including the bladder and prostate (32–34) (Figs. 11.21–11.24) (efigs 1138–1155). They can be asymptomatic or associated with hematuria, obstruction, or pelvic pain. SFT of the bladder presents as a submucosal mass that may be ulcerated. Microscopic features are identical to those seen at other sites, including spindle cells arranged in a haphazard or storiform pattern, zones of hypocellularity and hypercellularity, and deposition of intercellular dense collagen. Classic examples behave in a benign fashion if completely excised, although incompletely resected and unresectable cases recur locally. Malignant examples with cellular pleomorphism and high mitotic rate (greater than four per high-power field) have been described. Despite classic cytologic and growth pattern characteristics seen in most cases, even in TUR specimens, these tumors are commonly misdiagnosed as sarcoma or sarcomatoid carcinoma. Immunohistochemistry for CD34 and bcl-2 are positive in SFTs, aiding in their classification (33,34) (Table 11.1). Cytokeratins, epithelial membrane antigen, and smooth muscle markers are neg-

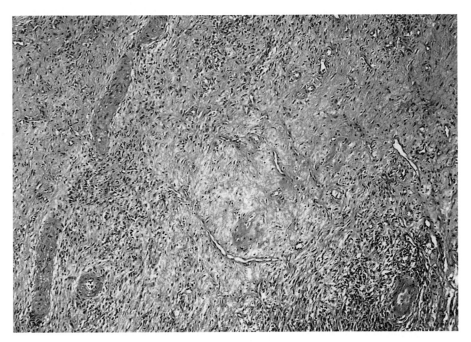

FIG. 11.21. Solitary fibrous tumor.

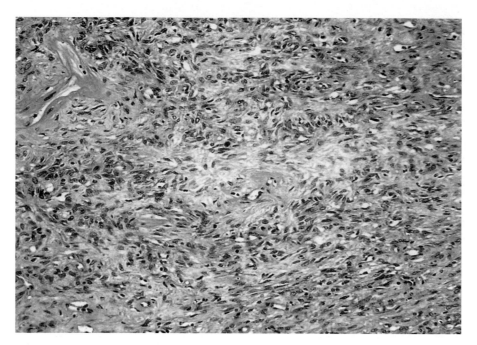

FIG. 11.22. Solitary fibrous tumor.

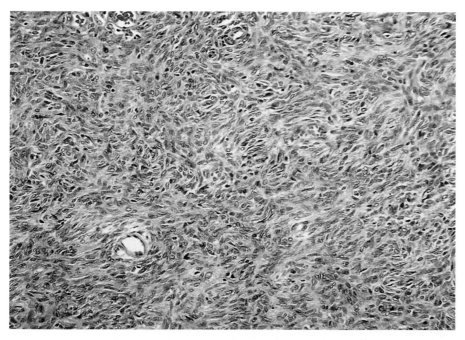

FIG. 11.23. Solitary fibrous tumor.

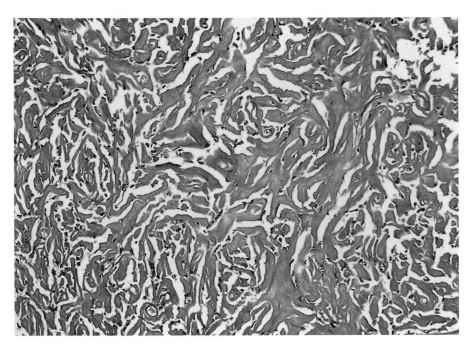

FIG. 11.24. Collagenized solitary fibrous tumor.

ative. Spindle cell tumors of dedicated prostatic stroma may secondarily involve the bladder and may also express these markers as well as progesterone receptors, the latter being negative in SFT.

MISCELLANEOUS MALIGNANT MESENCHYMAL TUMORS

Other sarcomas that have been described in the bladder include malignant fibrous histiocytoma (35,36), angiosarcoma (25,26), osteosarcoma (37), fibrosarcoma (38), and liposarcoma (39) (Fig. 11.25) (efigs 1156–1159). Even though it is possible for these tumors to arise in the bladder, it is more likely that they originate in other sites and involve the bladder secondarily. The possibility that these represent elements of heterologous differentiation in a sarcomatoid carcinoma should be ruled out by liberal sampling. We would consider tumors in patients with prior history of treated high-grade urothelial carcinoma with a predominant sarcoma histology as likely to have sarcomatoid carcinoma. The only exception is a patient treated with radiation therapy who develops a tumor 8 years or more after completing treatment. In this setting the tumor may represent a postradiation sarcoma.

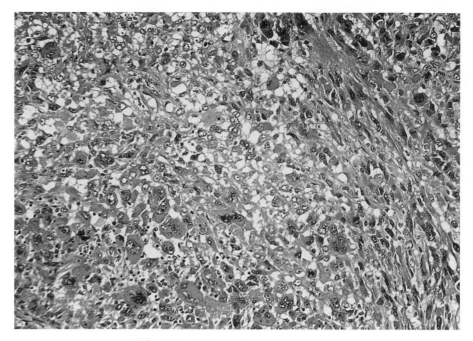

FIG. 11.25. Malignant fibrous histiocytoma.

REFERENCES

1. Mackenzie AR, Whitmore WF, Melamed MR. Myosarcomas of the bladder and prostate. *Cancer* 1968;22:833–844.
2. Russo P, Brady MS, Conlon K, et al. Adult urological sarcoma. *J Urol* 1992;147:1032–1037.
3. Weitzner S. Leiomyosarcoma of urinary bladder in children. *Urology* 1978;12:450–452.
4. Martin SA, Sears D, Sebo TJ, et al. Smooth muscle neoplasms of the urinary bladder. A clinicopathologic comparison of leiomyoma and leiomyosarcoma. *Am J Surg Pathol* 2002;26:292–300.
5. Lake MH, Kossow AS, Bokinsky G. Leiomyoma of the bladder and urethra. *J Urol* 1981;125: 742–743.
6. Yusim IE, Neulander EZ, Eidelberg I, et al. Leiomyoma of the genitourinary tract. *Scand J Urol Nephrol* 2001;35:295–299.
7. Swartz DA, Johnson DE, Ayala AG, et al. Bladder leiomyosarcoma: a review of 10 cases with five-year followup. *J Urol* 1985;1333:200–202.
8. Watanabe K, Baba A, Hoshi N, et al. Pseudosarcomatous myofibroblastic tumor and myosarcoma of the urogenital tract. Immunohistochemical characteristics and differential diagnosis. *Arch Pathol Lab Med* 2001;125:1070–1073.
9. Maurer HM. The intergroup rhabdomyosarcoma study (NIH). Objectives and clinical staging classification. *J Pediatr Surg* 1975;10:977–978.
10. Scholtmeijer RJ, Tromp CG, Hazebroeck FWJ. Embryonal rhabdomyosarcoma of the urogenital tract in childhood. *Eur Urol* 1983;9:69–74.
11. Hendricksson C, Zetterlund CG, Boisen P, et al. Large rhabdomyosarcoma of the urinary bladder in an adult. *Scand J Urol Nephrol* 1985;19:237–239.
12. Leuschner I, Harms D, Mattke A, et al. Rhabdomyosarcoma of the urinary bladder and vagina. A clinicopathologic study with emphasis on recurrent disease: a report from the Kiel pediatric tumor registry and the German CWS study. *Am J Surg Pathol* 2001;25:856–864.

13. Proppe KH, Scully RE, Rosai J. Postoperative spindle-cell nodules of the genitourinary tract resembling sarcomas: a report of eight cases. *Am J Surg Pathol* 1985;8:101–108.
14. Nochomovitz LE, Orenstein JM. Inflammatory pseudotumor of the urinary bladder—possible relationship to nodular fasciitis. *Am J Surg Pathol* 1985;9:366–373.
15. Jones EC, Clement PB, Young RH. Inflammatory pseudotumor of the urinary bladder. A clinicopathological, immunohistochemical, ultrastructural, and flow cytometric study of 13 cases. *Am J Surg Pathol* 1993;17:264–274.
16. Ro JY, Ayala AG, Ordonez NG, et al. Pseudosarcomatous fibromyxoid tumor of the urinary bladder. *Am J Clin Pathol* 1986;86:583–590.
17. Albores-Saavedra J, Manivel JC, Essenfeld H, et al. Pseudosarcomatous myofibroblastic proliferations in the urinary bladder of children. *Cancer* 1990;66:1234–1241.
18. Roth JA. Reactive pseudosarcomatous response in urinary bladder. *Urology* 1980;16:635–637.
19. Mahadevia PS, Alexander JE, Rojas-Corona R, et al. Pseudosarcomatous stromal reaction in primary and metastatic urothelial carcinoma: a source of diagnostic difficulty. *Am J Surg Pathol* 1989;13:782–790.
20. Wick MR, Brown BA, Young RH, et al. Spindle-cell proliferations of the urinary tract: an immunohistochemical study. *Am J Surg Pathol* 1988;12:379–389.
21. Reuter VE. Sarcomatoid lesions of the urogenital tract. *Semin Diag Pathol* 1993;10:188–201.
22. Young RH. Spindle cell lesions of the urinary tract. *Histol Histopathol* 1990;5:505–512.
23. Iczkowski KA, Shanks JH, Gadaleanu V, et al. Inflammatory pseudotumor and sarcoma of the urinary bladder: differential diagnosis and outcome in thirty-eight spindle cell neoplasms. *Mod Pathol* 2001;14:1043–1051.
24. Cook JR, Dehner LP, Collins MH, et al. Anaplastic lymphoma kinase (ALK) expression in inflammatory myofibroblastic tumor. *Am J Surg Pathol* 2001;25:1364–1371.
25. Fuleihan FM, Cordonnier JJ. Hemangioma of the bladder: report of a case and review of the literature. *J Urol* 1969;102:581–585.
26. Proca E. Haemangioma of the bladder. *Br J Urol* 1977;49:60.
27. Murao T, Kamoi M, Asano K. Fibroma of the bladder: a light and ultrastructural study of a case with review of the literature in Japan. *Acta Med Okayama* 1979;33:113–120.
28. Winfield HN, Catalona WJ. An isolated plexiform neurofibroma of the bladder. *J Urol* 1985;134:542–543.
29. Baumgartner G, Gaeta J, Wajsman Z, et al. Hemangiopericytoma of the urinary bladder: a case report and review of the literature. *J Surg Oncol* 1976;8:281–286.
30. Fletcher MS, Aker M, Hill JT, et al. Granular cell myoblastoma of the bladder. *Br J Urol* 1985;57:109–110.
31. Mouradian JA, Coleman JW, McGovern JH, et al. Granular cell tumor (myoblastoma) of the bladder. *J Urol* 1974;112:343–345.
32. Mentzel T, Bainbridge TC, Katenkamp D. Solitary fibrous tumor: clinicopathological, immunohistochemical, and ultrastructural analysis of 12 cases arising in soft tissues, nasal cavity and nasopharynx, urinary bladder and prostate. *Virchows Arch* 1997;430:445–453.
33. Westra WH, Grenko RT, Epstein J. Solitary fibrous tumor of the lower urogenital tract: a report of five cases involving the seminal vesicles, urinary bladder, and prostate. *Hum Pathol* 2000;31:63–68.
34. Corti B, Carella R, Gabusi E, et al. Solitary fibrous tumour of the urinary bladder with expression of bcl-2, CD34, and insulin-like growth factor type II. *Eur Urol* 2001;39:484–488.
35. Henriksen OB, Mogensen P, Engelholm AJ. Inflammatory fibrous histiocytoma of the bladder. *Acta Pathol Microbiol Immunol Scand (A)* 1982;90:333–337.
36. Turner AG. Malignant fibrous histiocytoma involving the bladder. *Br J Urol* 1985;57:237–238.
37. Berenson RJ, Flynn S, Freiha FS, et al. Primary osteogenic sarcoma of the bladder. *Cancer* 1986;57:350–355.
38. Foote JW, Seemayer TA, Duigan JP. Desmoid tumor involving the bladder: case report *J Urol* 1975;114:147–149.
39. Rosi P, Selli C, Carni M, et al. Myxoid liposarcoma of the bladder. *J Urol* 1983;130:560–561.

12

Miscellaneous Nontumors and Tumors

NONTUMORS

Amyloidosis

The bladder can be involved in cases of systemic amyloidosis but rarely is the primary site of this disease (1). The usual clinical presentation is that of hematuria. On cystoscopy, a localized amyloid tumor is seen as an elevated mass that can be confused with an invasive neoplasm. Less frequently, the disease may diffusely involve the bladder wall. Microscopically, the amyloid protein is an eosinophilic, afibrillar material deposited preferentially in the lamina propria and extending into the connective tissue surrounding muscle fascicles (2) (Fig. 12.1) (efigs 1160–1169). Less frequently, and usually in systemic amyloidosis, there are perivascular amyloid deposits. Congestion and hemorrhage are common but inflammatory cells are scanty unless the overlying epithelium is ulcerated. A few fibroblast-like cells are usually interspersed within the eosinophilic material. Special stains such as Congo red, crystal violet, or van Gieson helps establish the diagnosis. Patients with localized lesions are usually successfully managed by transurethral resection, but patients with more diffuse involvement may require more radical surgery to control bleeding (3).

Diverticular Disease

Bladder diverticula are relatively common yet their etiology remains controversial. Most investigators agree that they occur secondary to increased intravesical pressure as a result of obstruction distal to the diverticulum (4–6). The obstruction brings about compensatory muscle hypertrophy and eventual mucosal herniation in areas of weakness. Others believe that at least some diverticula are a consequence of congenital defects in the bladder musculature and they cite as evidence cases of diverticula in young patients without evidence of obstruction (7,8). The most common sites of diverticula are adjacent to the

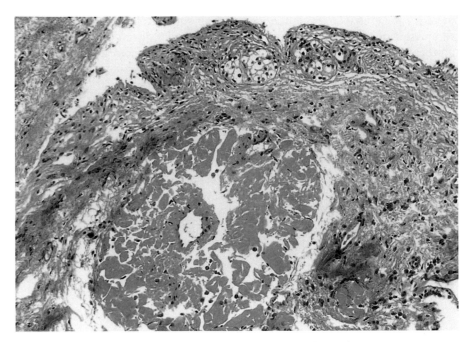

FIG. 12.1. Amyloidosis surrounding blood vessel.

ureteral orifices, the bladder dome (probably related to a urachal remnant), and the region of the internal urethral orifice. Grossly one sees distortion of the external surface of the bladder. The diverticula may be widely patent, but are usually narrow in symptomatic patients. The mucosa adjoining the diverticulum is usually hyperemic or ulcerated. There may be epithelial hyperplasia and the muscularis propria is hypertrophic. Commonly there is inflammation involving the lamina propria and muscularis propria. The wall of the diverticulum itself consists of urothelium and underlying connective tissue, similar to the bladder mucosa with lamina propria. In most cases of acquired diverticula, few, if any, muscle fascicles are identified. The true "congenital" diverticula contain a thinned outer muscle layer. Infrequently, the epithelium lining the sac undergoes squamous or glandular metaplasia resulting from local irritation associated with urine stasis, infection, or stone. In these cases it is not unusual for the diverticular wall to become extensively fibrotic.

Major complications of bladder diverticula include infection, lithiasis with subsequent obstruction, and carcinoma (9–11). It is believed that 2% to 7% of patients with bladder diverticula develop an associated neoplasm, which is thought to result from the chronic inflammatory stimuli mentioned earlier. The neoplasms may develop at the orifice or may occur within the diverticula, making endoscopic evaluation difficult. Whereas urothelial carcinomas predominate, there is a relative increase in the incidence of squamous carcinoma and adeno-carcinoma associated with squamous or glandular metaplasia in the lining urothelium. A distinct proclivity for clear cell adenocarcinomas of the bladder to occur in diverticula has been noted. Sarcomas and at least one carcinosarcoma also have been reported in association with bladder diverticula, but we believe that most of these cases represent sarcomatoid transformation in high-grade urothelial carcinomas (11).

Ectopic Prostatic Tissue

Ectopic prostatic polyps within the bladder are usually single, polypoid lesions around the trigone (12). These lesions typically present with gross and microscopic hematuria. The lesions may occur over a wide age range. Histolog-ically, the submucosal component of the urethral polyps is composed of stroma and prostatic glands (Fig. 12.2) (efigs 1170, 1171). The glands may be closely packed and in some areas may be cystically dilated at the periphery. The surface of urethral polyps is often papillary with broad papillae lined by urothelial cells, prostatic epithelial cells, or a combination of both. Rarely, these polyps have broad finger-like villous projections lined by benign prostatic epithelium. These lesions are benign.

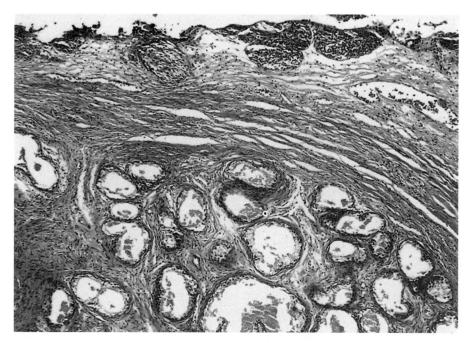

FIG. 12.2. Ectopic prostate tissue.

Pneumatosis

Rarely, air can be introduced into the bladder wall by high-pressure irrigation during cystoscopy, potentially leading to spontaneous bladder rupture. The situation is analogous to pneumatosis cystoides intestinalis (13) (Fig. 12.3) (efigs 1172–1174).

Fibroepithelial Polyp

Fibroepithelial polyp of the lower urinary tract is a relatively rare condition that is considered to be nonneoplastic, with some arising from acquired conditions and others congenitally (14). It has a marked male predominance. More than half of the reported cases occur in neonates or children; some cases are associated with urogenital malformations. However, cases have also been reported in patients in their second to fourth decades. The main clinical manifestations are urinary obstruction, urinary hesitancy, dysuria, enuresis, hematuria, infection, and flank pain. Fibroepithelial polyps are usually diagnosed by cystourethrography or cystoscopy and are treated by transurethral resection, following which the lesion does not usually recur. Most cases are located near the verumontanum or the bladder neck. Histologically, fibroepithelial polyps are predominantly composed of urothelial epithelium and fibrovascular stroma

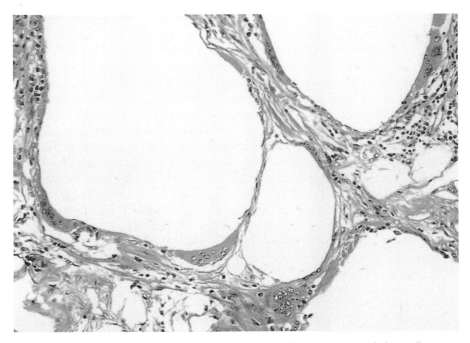

FIG. 12.3. Pneumatosis with air spaces surrounded by multinucleated giant cells.

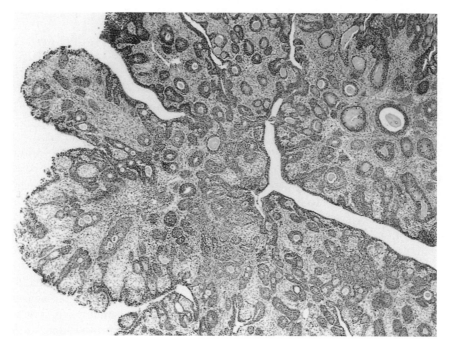

FIG. 12.4. Fibroepithelial polyp.

showing a finger-like or polypoid growth pattern (Figs. 12.4–12.6) (efigs 1175–1180). Urothelium shows tubular or anastomosing structures with colloid-like secretions in some cases, resembling cystitis glandularis. Although some urothelium shows focal squamous or mucinous metaplasia or becomes thin or denuded, none contain any cytologic atypia. The stroma of the polyps typically contains relatively frequent small vessels, some of which were dilated or congested. Stromal edema, either focal or extensive, is also a common finding. Although the stromal cells can show atypia with multinucleated cells and hyperchromasia, the atypia appears degenerative in nature, lacking prominent nucleoli and mitoses.

Urothelial papilloma may be difficult to differentiate from fibroepithelial polyp because both lesions show a polypoid or finger-like growth pattern and lack of cytologic atypia of the urothelium. However, urothelial papilloma usually has thin fibrovascular cores in contrast to the relatively broad stroma of fibroepithelial polyp.

FIG. 12.6. Fibroepithelial polyp.

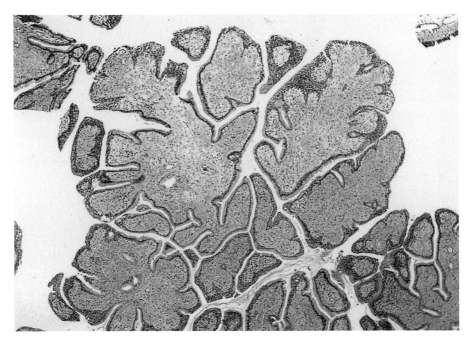

FIG. 12.5. Fibroepithelial polyp.

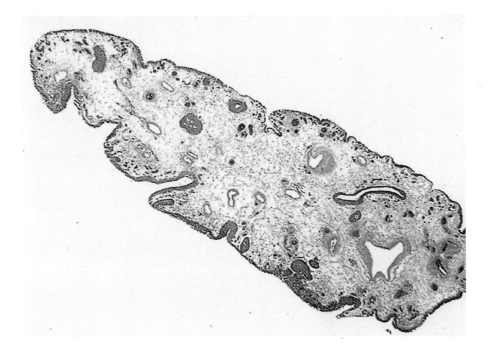

TUMORS

Paraganglioma

Of paragangliomas throughout the body, 10% occur in extraadrenal sites; of these extraadrenal tumors, 10% are found in the bladder wall (15,16). Paragangliomas of the urinary bladder account for less than 0.5% of bladder tumors. Primary paragangliomas of the bladder, which have also been designated as bladder pheochromocytomas, have a female-to-male ratio of 3:2 with an average age diagnosis of 41 years. There is a wide age distribution from childhood to older age. Most tumors are located either on the dome or trigone. Although most patients have exophytic lesions with intact mucosa, some patients have ulceration of the overlying mucosa. Lesions vary greatly in size from 2 mm to 10 cm. Most patients present with solitary lesions.

Paragangliomas can often be diagnosed on clinical grounds. Seventy-five percent of patients experience micturition attacks. When the bladder fills or upon urination, there ensues bursts of headaches, palpitations, hypertension, blurred vision, sweating, anxiety, tremulousness, and sometimes syncope. Hypertension can also be induced by intraoperative manipulation of the tumor. Hematuria is found in 60% of patients, whereas dysuria is uncommon. Increases in serum or urine catecholamines can provide laboratory confirmation of the diagnosis.

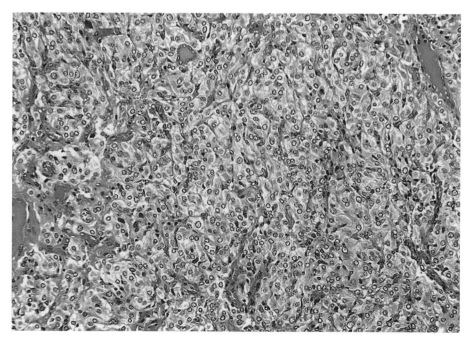

FIG. 12.7. Paraganglioma.

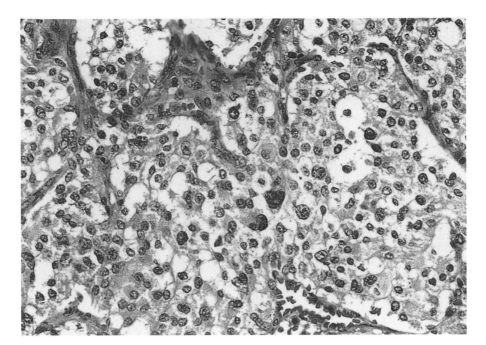

FIG. 12.8. Paraganglioma.

Radiologically, bladder paragangliomas may be diagnosed using arteriography, selective venous sampling, computed tomography, magnetic resonance imaging, and scintigraphy with meta-^{131}I iodobenzyoguanidine (^{131}I-MIBG).

Paragangliomas typically are composed of nests (Zellballen) separated by either a thin delicate plexiform vascular network or more fibrous septa (Figs. 12.7, 12.8) (efigs 1181–1194). At higher magnification, polyhedric cells have acidophilic to amphophilic cytoplasm with central or eccentric nuclei and visible nucleoli. As in many endocrine tumors, occasional bizarre nuclei may be seen (Fig. 12.9). Their chromatin appears smudged and hyperchromatic without mitoses, typical of degenerative atypia rather than the atypia of a high-grade malignant tumor. Mitoses may be present yet are usually not numerous. Paragangliomas of the bladder can invade deeply into the muscle or show vascular invasion. Focal hemorrhage and necrosis may also be present. Occasionally, one can discern neuroblastic or ganglioneuromatous differentiation. Cases of paraganglioma of the urinary bladder have been described in patients with neurofibromatosis. Invasive urothelial carcinoma on occasion grow in a nesting pattern reminiscent of paraganglioma (Figs. 12.10, 12.11). However, these urothelial tumors are likely to be associated with carcinoma in situ or noninvasive papillary carcinoma, whereas the urothelium overlying a paraganglioma is normal, reactive, or ulcerated. In contrast to pheochromocytomas, urothelial carcinomas

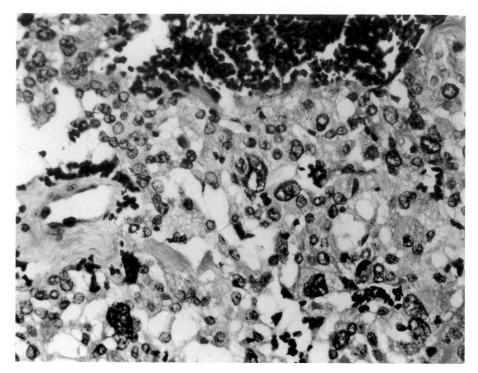

FIG. 12.9. Paraganglioma with degenerative atypia.

exhibit cytologic atypia consisting of enlarged nuclei, prominent nucleoli, and numerous mitotic figures. Furthermore, the nesting and vascular pattern in urothelial carcinoma tends to be only focally present. In cases in which the authors have seen paragangliomas misdiagnosed as urothelial carcinoma, the major histologic features that led to the incorrect diagnosis included a diffuse growth pattern, focal clear cells, necrosis, and muscularis propria invasion, with significant cautery artifact compounding the diagnostic problems (17). Distinction between paraganglioma and urothelial cancer is critical because of different therapeutic options, with paragangliomas treated by transurethral resection of bladder or partial cystectomy.

Paragangliomas usually react with antisera to neuron-specific enolase (NSE), synaptophysin, and chromogranin and are negative with antibodies to various keratins. Immunostains for S-100 show sustentacular cells surrounding tumor nests. In contrast, invasive urothelial carcinomas are positive for CK7, CK20, and high-molecular-weight cytokeratin. Poorly differentiated urothelial carcino-

FIG. 12.11. Invasive urothelial carcinoma with nested pattern resembling paraganglioma.

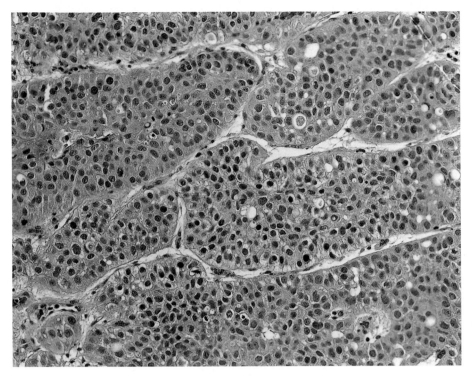

FIG. 12.10. Invasive urothelial carcinoma with nested pattern resembling paraganglioma.

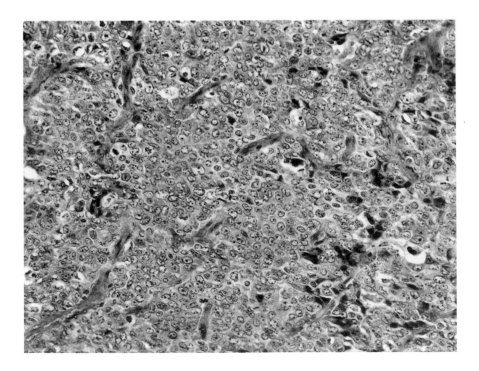

mas can also show NSE immunoreactivity. Urothelial carcinomas have not been systematically studied for chromogranin. Cases of melanin-containing pigmented paragangliomas within the bladder have been reported.

No histologic criteria (e.g., atypia, vascular invasion, size, muscle invasion) are predictive of which lesions are capable of distant spread. Only those tumors that have metastasized may be confidently diagnosed as malignant. Approximately 10% to 15% of paragangliomas of the bladder are malignant. Most local metastases are to the iliohypogastric lymph nodes with distant spread most commonly to the lung. Localized tumors are treated by transurethral resection, wedge resection, or partial cystectomy. Treatment for malignant paraganglioma of the bladder is radical cystectomy with removal of metastases if possible. Radiation and chemotherapy appear to have limited effectiveness. Ancillary studies, such as DNA ploidy, p53 expression, and proliferation (MIB-1 labeling), do not appear predictive of clinical outcome. In one large series, a better prognosis was seen in patients with stage T1 or T2 tumors that were completely resected.

Paragangliomas of the bladder most likely arise from paraganglia that may uncommonly be found in the bladder neck smooth muscle (18) (Fig. 12.12) (Color Plate 15) (efigs 1195–1202). Rarely, paraganglia may be seen on transurethral resection (TUR) or on needle biopsy where their distinction from carcinoma must be made. These consist of clusters of clear or amphophilic cells

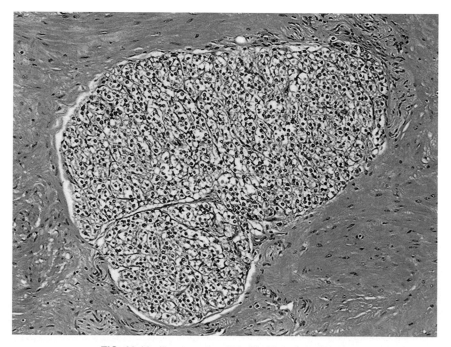

FIG. 12.12. Paraganglia within bladder musculature.

with fine cytoplasmic granules and a prominent vascular pattern, often intimately related to nerves. Nucleoli are not prominent; if nuclear atypia is present, it is degenerative in appearance as seen in endocrine lesions. Verification of the diagnosis can be accomplished with positive immunostaining for neuroendocrine markers and for S-100 in sustentacular cells.

Hematologic Malignancies

Lymphomas involving the bladder have a female tendency with most reported cases in middle-aged women (19,20). Tumors may be classified as (a) primary localized in the bladder, (b) presenting in the bladder as the first sign of systemic disease, and (c) recurrent in patients with a history of malignant lymphoma (secondary lymphoma). Primary lymphomas localized to the bladder are rare, accounting for only between 0.15% and 2% of all extranodal lymphomas. Most are B-cell non-Hodgkin lymphoma, with the most common subtype being MALT-type lymphoma. Lymphoepithelial lesions are found in only a minority of reported bladder MALT-type lymphomas. Lymphomas presenting in the bladder and secondary lymphomas are predominantly of large cell type (efigs 1203, 1204). Other subtypes of lymphomas have been reported in the bladder, often as case reports, with follicular small-cleaved types being relatively more represented (Fig. 12.13) (efigs 1205–1208). Patients typically present nonspecifically

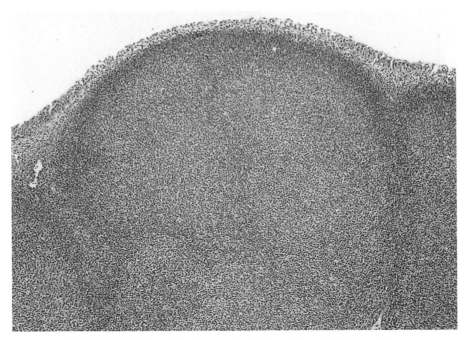

FIG. 12.13. Malignant lymphoma, small cleaved type, follicular pattern.

with hematuria and sometimes with frequency and dysuria. Urine cytology is typically not diagnostic and a tissue biopsy is required. Grossly, lymphomatous lesions of the bladder appear as solitary submucosal masses, although they may be multifocal. The urothelium is typically intact, although ulceration has been recorded. Treatment typically consists of transurethral resection followed by chemotherapy or radiotherapy. Prognosis depends on the type of lymphoma present, with MALT-type lymphomas having a good prognosis with a tendency to remain localized to the bladder for a long time and with low risk of dissemination. On the other hand, diffuse large cell lymphomas have a more aggressive course. Patients with recurrent lymphoma have the worst prognosis, often measured in months, because it is a sign of widely disseminated disease resistant to therapy. When presented with an undifferentiated tumor within the bladder, the presumption may be that it is an undifferentiated carcinoma, given that the overwhelming majority of bladder tumors are carcinomas. Immunohistochemical stains for epithelial and lymphoid markers should be performed in this setting.

The bladder is a rare site of primary plasmacytoma (21) (Fig. 12.14) (efigs 1209–1211). Care must be taken to exclude urothelial carcinoma with plasmacytoid features. Immunohistochemical stains for keratin and kappa and lambda light chains can help resolve the differential diagnosis. Most patients with extramedullary plasmacytoma are adults with nonspecific symptoms of hema-

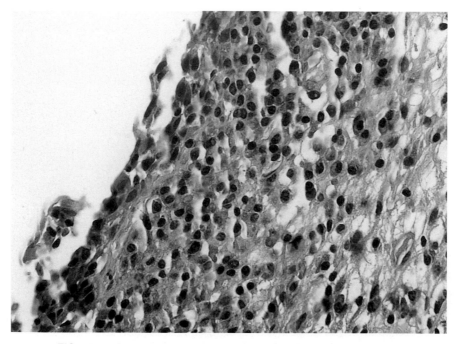

FIG. 12.14. Plasmacytoma (cells showed lambda light chain restriction).

turia and dysuria. Although the lesions may be diffusely infiltrative, they tend to form intraluminal masses. Patients who have been treated with cystectomy have had excellent results, although extramedullary plasmacytomas in other sites are typically treated with radiotherapy.

REFERENCES

1. Malek RS, Greene LF, Farrow GM. Amyloidosis of the urinary bladder. *Br J Urol* 1971;43:189–200.
2. Farah RN, Benson DO, Fine G, et al. Primary localized amyloidosis of bladder. *Urology* 1979;13: 200–202.
3. Akhtar M, Valencia M, Thomas AM. Solitary primary amyloidosis of urinary bladder. *Urology* 1978;12:721–724.
4. Miller A. The aetiology and treatment of diverticulum of the bladder. *Br J Urol* 1958;30:43–56.
5. Kertsschmer HL. Diverticula of the urinary bladder. A clinical study of 236 cases. *Surg Gynecol Obstet* 1940;71:491–503.
6. Fox M, Power RF, Bruce AW. Diverticulum of the bladder. Presentation and evaluation of treatment of 115 cases. *Br J Urol* 1962;34:286–298.
7. Schiff M, Lytton B. Congenital diverticulum of the bladder. *J Urol* 1970;104:111–115.
8. Barrett DW, Malek RS, Kelalis PP. Observations on vesical diverticulum in childhood. *J Urol* 1976;116:234–236.
9. Abeshouse BS, Goldstein AE. Primary carcinoma in a diverticulum of the bladder. A report of four cases and a review of the literature. *J Urol* 1943;49:534–547.
10. Faysal MH, Freiha FS. Primary neoplasia in vesical diverticula: a report of 12 cases. *Br J Urol* 1978; 53:141–143.
11. Ward MP. Sarcoma of vesical diverticula. *Br J Urol* 1958;30:57–59.
12. Remick DG, Kumar NB. Benign polyps with prostatic-type epithelium of urethra and the urinary bladder. *Am J Surg Pathol* 1984;8:833–839.
13. Kravchick S, Cytron S, Lobik L, et al. Clot retention and spontaneous rupture with secondary pneumatosis of bladder wall following routine cystoscopy. *Pathol Oncol Res* 2001;7:301–302.
14. Young RH: Fibroepithelial polyp of the bladder with atypical stromal cells. *Arch Pathol Lab Med* 1986;110:241–242.
15. Cheng L, Leibovich BC, Cheville JC, et al. Paraganglioma of the urinary bladder: Can biologic potential be predicted? *Cancer* 2000;88:844–852.
16. Nakatani T, Hayama T, Uchida J, et al. Diagnostic localization of extra-adrenal pheochromocytoma: comparison of [123] I-MIBG imaging and [131] I-MIBG imaging. *Oncol Rep* 2002;9:1225–1227.
17. Zhou M, Epstein JI, Young RH. Paraganglioma of the urinary bladder: a lesion often misdiagnosed as urothelial carcinoma in transurethral resection specimens. *Am J Surg Pathol* (in press).
18. Ostrowski ML, Wheeler TM. Paraganglia of the prostate: location, frequency, and differentiation from prostatic adenocarcinoma. *Am J Surg Pathol* 1994;18:412–420.
19. Wazait HD, Chahal R, Sundurum SK, et al. MALT-type primary lymphoma of the urinary bladder: clinicopathological study of 2 cases and review of the literature. *Urol Int* 2001;66:220–224.
20. Kempton CL, Kurtin PJ, Inwards DJ, et al. Malignant lymphoma of the bladder: evidence from 36 cases that low-grade lymphoma of the MALT-type is the most common primary bladder lymphoma. *Am J Surg Pathol* 1997;21:1324–1333.
21. Ho DS, Patterson AL, Orozco RE, et al. Extramedullary plasmacytoma of the bladder: case report and review of the literature. *J Urol* 1993;150:473–474.

13

Secondary Tumors of the Bladder

The bladder may be involved secondarily by tumors from adjacent sites such as the prostate, seminal vesicles, lower intestinal tract, and the female genital tract (1,2). Tumors may involve the bladder by direct extension or metastasis. The diagnostic problems posed for the pathologist in cases of secondary involvement vary according to the morphology of the primary neoplasm; for example, female genital tract tumors or anal canal tumors with squamous cell carcinoma histology may mimic or may be impossible to distinguish from a primary bladder tumor. In most cases, however, clinical features aid in the diagnosis. Uncommon metastatic tumors to the bladder that enter the differential diagnosis of different types and variants of bladder carcinoma include malignant melanoma (with plasmacytoid variant), metastatic renal cell carcinoma (with urothelial carcinoma with clear cell change and clear cell adenocarcinoma) and metastatic small cell carcinoma (3–6). A common differential diagnostic dilemma of a poorly differentiated carcinoma in transurethral resections of the bladder or prostate is the distinction between high-grade invasive urothelial carcinoma and a poorly differentiated prostatic adenocarcinoma. The presence of squamous differentiation, urothelial carcinoma in situ (CIS), and high degree of nuclear anaplasia favor the diagnosis of urothelial carcinoma. Prostate carcinomas that are poorly differentiated may have a more diffuse growth, with only focal evidence of glandular differentiation. In these instances, the tumor cells are usually more homogeneous with prominent nucleoli. A clinical history and assistance with immunohistochemical stains [prostate-specific antigen (PSA) and prostate-specific acid phosphatase (PSAP)] are important. Thrombomodulin, p63, or high-molecular-weight cytokeratin stains are also useful in a panel as positive markers for urothelial carcinomas (7).

The bladder may be involved secondarily by direct extension of a tumor from adjacent viscera (such as the prostate, cervix, or rectum) or less commonly by a metastatic tumor from a distant site. Malignant lymphoma or leukemia may also secondarily involve the bladder as part of a more disseminated or systemic manifestation (see Chapter 12). Finally, patients with urothelial carcinoma of the upper tract (pelvicalyceal system or ureter) or lower tract (urethra) may subsequently develop bladder cancer.

TUMORS INVOLVING THE BLADDER BY DIRECT EXTENSION

Carcinomas of the cervix, rectosigmoid, and prostate account for the most common primary neoplasms involving the bladder by direct extension, although other cancers such as those from the endometrium, ovary, appendix, and other segments of the colon may involve the bladder (8,9) Figs. 13.1–13.4) (efigs 1212–1226). The extent of diagnostic problems posed by secondary involvement depends on the morphology of the primary tumor. Müllerian tumors for the most part have sufficiently distinctive histology to enable them to be recognized as secondary tumors. The exceptions are clear cell carcinoma from the endometrium or ovary and mucinous carcinoma of the ovary or appendix with enteric morphology. In these cases, it is essential to determine the pattern of involvement (whether a tumor involves the bladder from "outside in") and correlate findings with imaging studies and clinicopathologic findings. Distinction of a squamous cell carcinoma (primary cervix, anal canal, or bladder) and enteric adenocarcinoma (primary rectosigmoid or bladder) requires similar attention to patterns of involvement and correlation with imaging and operative findings to arrive at the appropriate diagnosis. On the basis of morphology alone, these distinctions are difficult, if not impossible. Direct extension from the prostate is often easy to recognize because of the frequent nuclear monotony and acinar differentiation in prostate cancer (Figs. 13.5–13.8) (efigs

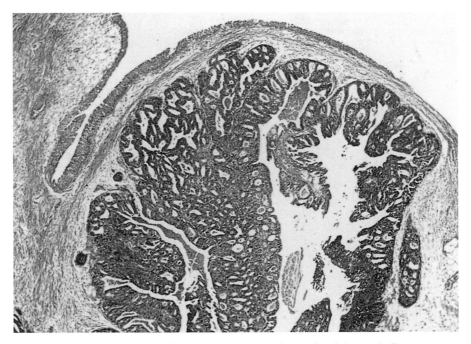

FIG. 13.1. Metastatic adenocarcinoma from colon undermining urothelium.

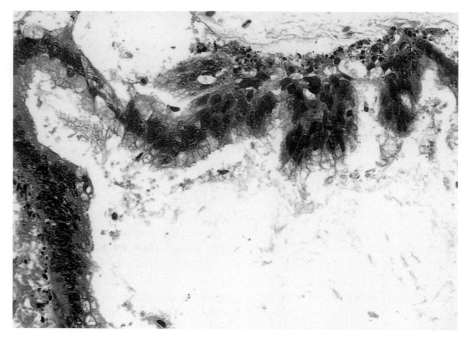

FIG. 13.2. Metastatic adenocarcinoma from colon (higher magnification of Figure 13.1).

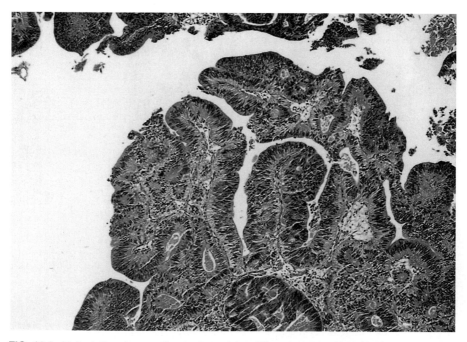

FIG. 13.3. Metastatic adenocarcinoma from colon. When tumor reaches bladder luminal surface, it develops papillary fronds mimicking primary adenocarcinoma of the bladder.

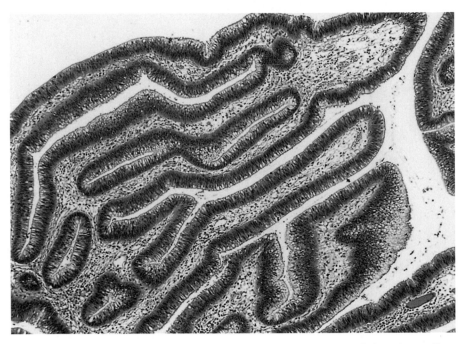

FIG. 13.4. Metastatic adenocarcinoma from colon. In some areas, tumor mimics primary villous adenoma of bladder.

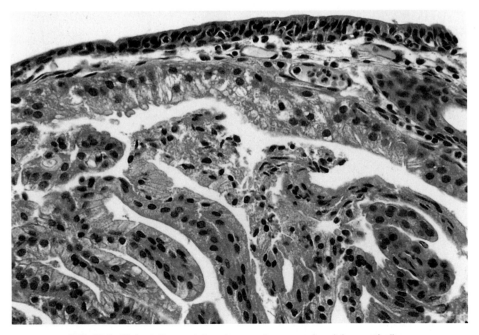

FIG. 13.5. Metastatic prostate adenocarcinoma undermining urothelium.

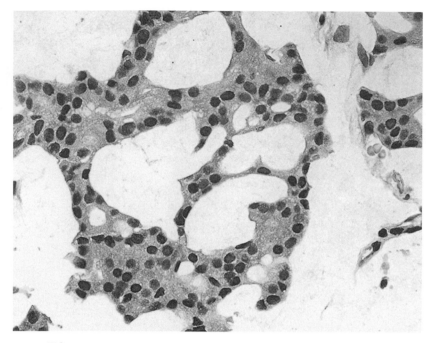

FIG. 13.6. Metastatic prostate adenocarcinoma with mucinous features.

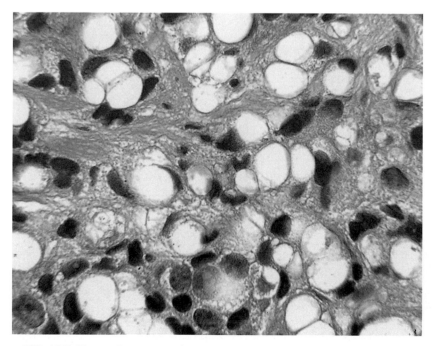

FIG. 13.7. Metastatic prostate adenocarcinoma with signet ring–like cell features.

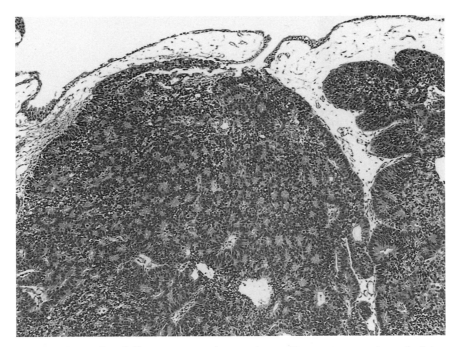

FIG. 13.8. Metastatic cribriform prostate adenocarcinoma. Tumor merges onto urothelial surface.

1227–1239). If prostate cancer has a more sheetlike growth, the histology of the bladder can be mimicked. Conversely, bladder cancer with predominantly clear cell histology can mimic prostate cancer. Immunohistochemical stains (PSA and PSAP, which are positive in prostate cancer; thrombomodulin, high-molecular-weight cytokeratin, and p63, which are positive in urothelial cancer) are helpful (7).

METASTASIS TO THE BLADDER

Comprehensive autopsy studies show that several carcinomas from diverse primary sites can metastasize to the bladder. These sites include the stomach, colon, pancreas, breast, and lung (more common primaries), as well as other less common primary sites such as the kidney, testis, gallbladder, liver, and tongue (3,5,10–12). In general, metastasis should be suspected when there is an absence of a mucosal abnormality (urothelial or glandular CIS or a mucosal based mass), frequent vascular invasion, involvement of muscularis propria only, or a histology not conforming to the commonly encountered histologic patterns of bladder cancer.

Particular problems are posed with carcinoma with signet ring cell histology (stomach, breast, and prostate versus bladder), plasmacytoid histology

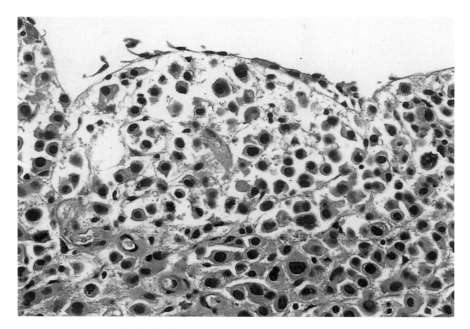

FIG. 13.9. Metastatic adenocarcinoma from breast.

(melanoma and lymphoma versus bladder carcinoma), clear cell histology (kidney and prostate versus bladder), small cell histology (lung and other viscera versus bladder), and enteric histology [colon, ovary, appendix, and prostate (ductal) versus bladder] (Fig. 13.9) (Color Plates 16) (efigs 1240–1249).

Distinction of a metastasis from the colon versus a bladder primary (primary adenocarcinoma and urothelial carcinoma with enteric differentiation) is difficult to impossible, because metastatic colonic tumors can even involve the mucosa and secondarily colonize it to create a villous architecture that would suggest a primary bladder tumor (13,14) (efigs 1212–1226). The presence of widespread intestinal metaplasia and chronic bladder disease favor a bladder primary. Urothelial carcinoma with enteric differentiation may show obvious conventional urothelial carcinoma histology or urothelial CIS. In the absence of these factors, distinction from a metastasis is not tenable on morphologic grounds. A history of high-grade, high-stage colon cancer is important and, if present, an adenocarcinoma in the bladder with enteric histology should be considered as a metastasis. Immunohistochemical or histochemical studies assessing mucin or cytokeratin subtypes are not useful. A recent study suggests that beta catenin is present on immunohistochemistry in cases of a colonic primary and is absent in primary bladder adenocarcinoma (15).

REFERENCES

1. Melicow MM. Tumors of the urinary bladder: a clinicopathological analysis of over 2500 specimens and biopsies. *J Urol* 1955;74:498–521.
2. Young RH, Johnston WH. Serous adenocarcinoma of the uterus metastatic to the urinary bladder mimicking primary bladder neoplasia: a report of a case. *Am J Surg Pathol* 1990;14:877–880.
3. Sim SJ, Ro JY, Ordonez NG, et al. Metastatic renal cell carcinoma to the bladder: a clinicopathologic and immunohistochemical study. *Mod Pathol* 1999;12:351–355.
4. Oliva E, Amin MB, Jimenez R, et al. Clear cell carcinoma of the urinary bladder: a report and comparison of four tumors of mullerian origin and nine of probable urothelial origin with discussion of histogenesis and diagnostic problems. *Am J Surg Pathol* 2002;26:190–197.
5. Matsuo M, Koga S, Nishikido M, et al. Renal cell carcinoma with solitary metachronous metastasis to the urinary bladder. *Urology* 2002;60:911–912.
6. Coltart RS, Stewart S, Brown CH. Small cell carcinoma of the bronchus: a rare cause of haematuria from a metastasis in the urinary bladder. *J R Soc Med* 1985;78:1053–1054.
7. Varma M, Morgan M, Amin MB, et al. High molecular weight cytokeratin antibody (clone 34betaE12): a sensitive marker for differentiation of high-grade invasive urothelial carcinoma from prostate cancer. *Histopathology* 2003;42:167–172.
8. Klinger ME. Secondary tumors of the genito-urinary tract. *J Urol* 1951;65:144–153.
9. Henry R, Bracken RB, Ayala A. Appendiceal carcinoma mimicking primary bladder cancer. *J Urol* 1980;123:590–591.
10. Van Driel MF, Ypma AFGVM, Van Gelder B. Gastric carcinoma metastatic to the bladder. *Brit J Urol* 1987;59:193–194.
11. Silverstein LI, Plaine L, Davis JE, et al. Breast carcinoma metastatic to bladder. *Urology* 1987;29:544–547.
12. Chalbaud RA, Johnson DE. Adenocarcinoma of tongue metastatic to bladder. *Urology* 1974;4:454–455.
13. Silver SA, Epstein JI. Adenocarcinoma of the colon simulating primary urinary bladder neoplasia. A report of nine cases. *Am J Surg Pathol* 1993;17:171–178.
14. Tamboli P, Mohsin SK, Hailemariam S, et al. Colonic adenocarcinoma metastatic to the urinary tract versus primary tumors of the urinary tract with glandular differentiation: a report of 7 cases and investigation using a limited immunohistochemical panel. *Arch Pathol Lab Med* 2002;126:1057–1063.
15. Wang HL, Lu DW, Yerian LM, et al. Immunohistochemical distinction between primary adenocarcinoma of the bladder and secondary colorectal adenocarcinoma. *Am J Surg Pathol* 2001;25:1380–1387.

Subject Index